THE COMPLETE KETOGENIC DIET COOKBOOK

KETO BREAD & KETO FAT BOMB

150+ Instantly Amazing Savory & Sweet, Frozen & Liquid Snacks Recipes for Busy People on Paleo, Gluten-Free, Low-Carb & Ketogenic Diet

SANDRA M.

ISBN: 9781792828225

TABLE OF CONTENT

Introduction

I want to thank you and congratulate you for purchasing the book, **"THE COMPLETE KETOGENIC DIET COOKBOOK: KETO BREAD & KETO FAT BOMB – 150+ Instantly Amazing Savory & Sweet, Frozen & Liquid Snacks Recipes for Busy People on Paleo, Gluten-Free, Low-Carb & Ketogenic Diet "**

In recent years, the ketogenic diet, or keto diet, has been known by the millions of people around the world. The ketogenic diet is a high fat, low carb, and moderate proteins diet that makes the body change its energy source from the use of glucose supplied from sugar and carbohydrates to the use of fat for energy in a process known as ketosis. When this state is established, your body will burn fat, instead of glucose, for energy needs.

The ketogenic diet is one of the easiest diets to follow because you get to eat bacon, butter, meat, avocado and others kinds of high- fat food, But at the same time, you also are not allowed to eat certain types of food too as Fruit, Grains and Starches, Root Vegetables, Some Oils, Low-Fat Dairy, Sweetened Sauces and Dips, Grain Products.

The ketogenic diet allows you to see results within the first few days and easily make you to the changes new your lifestyle for fast and effective weight loss way

Keto fat bomb and Keto bread is part of the ketogenic diet.

Fat bombs, also called keto bombs, are simply energy balls or protein balls with ingredients low protein, high fat and no sugar such as butter, coconut oil, butter cheese, avocados ... that you can eat on desserts, snacks or other meals replacement. They are simple and easy to make and extremely satisfying to eat.

And with keto bread, you can still make it when using others ingredient that is keto friendly, instead of conventional wheat flour for the ketogenic diet process. The most important thing you need to know is what to substitute for wheat flour. The recipes use almond flour, coconut flour, or even cauliflower. And then you can still eat your favorite staples like bread, muffins, pancakes, waffles, pizzas, crackers, bagels, buns, and breadsticks.

This cookbook contains over healthy 150 Ketogenic recipes, includes savory & sweet food, with frozen & liquid, on keto fat bombs and keto bread recipes. They are simple and easy to make and extremely satisfying to eat. That is suitable not only for the ketogenic diet or gluten-free but also the low carb and paleo diets. That will help your weight loss and also help you in adopting a healthier lifestyle.

Thank again for purchasing this book, I hope to enjoy it!

Chapter 1: THE BASIC KNOWLEDGE ABOUT KETOGENIC DIET

What is Weight Loss

Weight loss is the weight that you lose when your body undergoes a process of what the experts term as a caloric deficiency. This can be achieved either by boosting your calories requirement through the building of muscle mass while keeping your intake constant or via calorie restriction in the form of a diet where your daily calorie intake is designed to be lesser than your daily requirement.

When your body finds itself in a state where calories input is lesser than what it needs to daily function, it will seek to get energy from stores of energy within your body. Most of the time these would be from the stores of glucose found in the liver as well as from your muscle. The other major energy store found in our body would be the fats that we carry on our frame. This is where the tricky part comes in. If your body isn't conditioned for burning fats, it will quickly use up the glucose stores, and that is when the feeling of hunger will come into potentially derail you from your weight loss mission

What is the Ketogenic Diet?

The Ketogenic diet (also known as keto diet or "nutritional ketosis") is a high- fat, adequate-protein, low-carbohydrate diet. It reduces the amount of sugar and insulin in the blood and causes the body's metabolism to switch from carb to fat and ketones.

The ketogenic diet is an effective tool for weight loss because of the dramatic decrease in carb intake, forcing your body to burn fat instead of carbs for energy.

On a ketogenic diet, your entire body switches its fuel supply to run almost entirely on fat. Insulin levels become very low, and fat burning increases dramatically. It becomes easy to access your fat stores to burn them off. This is great if you're trying to lose weight, but there are also other less obvious benefits, such as less hunger and a steady supply of energy, keeping you alert and focused.

When the body produces ketones, it's said to be in ketosis. The fastest way to get there is by fasting – not eating anything – but nobody can fast forever.

A keto diet, on the other hand, can be eaten indefinitely and also results in ketosis. It has many of the benefits of fasting – including weight loss – without having to fast.

Your daily intake of carb is only limited to 20g of carb - that is extremely low. This means you can not eat bread, biscuits, rice, starchy vegetables, most fruits or any kind of sugar.

However, with the Keto diet, you can comfortably eat fatty foods like butter, cheese, cream, nuts, and even bacon. You can also eat a variety of different types of protein, lots of green leafy vegetables and vegetables like cucumber, pepper, onion, tomato, broccoli, and cauliflower.

Ketosis

The "keto" in a ketogenic diet comes from the fact that it makes the body produce small fuel molecules called "ketones". This is a alternative fuel for the body, used when blood sugar (glucose) is in short supply.

Ketones are produced if you eat very few carbs (that are quickly broken down into blood sugar) and only moderate amounts of protein (excess protein can also be converted to blood sugar).

Ketones are produced in the liver, from fat. They are then used as fuel throughout the body, including the brain. The brain is a hungry organ that consumes lots of energy every day, and it can't run on fat directly. It can only run on glucose… or ketones.

On a ketogenic diet, your entire body switches its fuel supply to run almost entirely on fat. Insulin levels become very low, and fat burning increases dramatically. It becomes easy to access your fat stores to burn them off. This is great if you're trying to lose weight, but there are also other less obvious benefits, such as less hunger and a steady supply of energy, keeping you alert and focused.

When the body produces ketones, it's said to be in ketosis. The fastest way to get there is by fasting – not eating anything – but nobody can fast forever.

A keto diet, on the other hand, can be eaten indefinitely and also results in ketosis. It has many of the benefits of fasting – including weight loss – without having to fast.

Ketones

Ketones are the metabolic fuel produced when your body shifts into fat-burning mode.

Glucose and ketones are the only energy sources used by the brain. Think of ketones as the auxiliary power source of your body.

Before the advent of agriculture, when our ancestors were hunter-gatherers, they fasted regularly. When food was scarce, they didn't have a choice but to wait for for an opportune time to hunt for food and cook it.

They had a very low intake of carbs and protein and thus were unintentionally running on ketones. Converting stored fat into energy is hardwired for our survival and a natural part of human existence.

Your body burns fat to use and produce ketones whenever glucose sources are low or depleted, such as:

- during fasting,

- after prolonged exercise

- when you eat a ketogenic diet.

Lipase (an enzyme responsible for fat breakdown) releases stored triglycerides (fats). These fatty acids go to your liver and your liver turns them into ketones.

There are three types of ketone bodies:

- Acetoacetate – During the breakdown of long- and medium-chain fatty acids for energy, acetoacetate is produced first.

• Acetone – Spontaneously, acetone is also produced as a by-product of acetoacetate. Both of these ketone bodies, when not used, spill into your urine and breath, making urine and breath testing a promising measurement of whether or not you're going into ketosis. More on this below in How to Test Ketone Levels.

• Beta-hydroxybutyrate (BHB) – Not technically a ketone but a molecule. Its essential role in the ketogenic diet makes it counts as the important ketone body. BHB is synthesized by your liver from acetoacetate. BHB is important because it can freely float throughout your body in your blood, crossing many tissues where other molecules can't. It enters the mitochondria and gets turned into ATP (adenosine triphosphate), the energy currency of your cells. BHB = ATP = energy!

Now that you know what ketones are and how ketosis works, you probably want to know why you should consider eating a ketogenic diet — the diet that promotes ketosis.

Keto and weight loss

Turning your body into a fat-burning machine has obvious benefits for weight loss. Fat burning is vastly increased, while insulin – the fat-storing hormone – levels drop greatly. This creates ideal circumstances in which fat loss can occur, without hunger.

More than 30 high-quality scientific studies show that, compared to other diets, low-carb and keto diets result in more effective weight loss.

Appetite control

On keto, you'll gain a new control over your appetite. When your body burns fat 24-7, it has constant access to weeks or months of stored energy, dramatically reducing feelings of hunger. It's a very common experience, and studies prove it.

This makes it easy to eat less and lose excess weight – just don't eat until you're hungry. This makes intermittent fasting easy, super-charging efforts to reverse type 2 diabetes and speeding up weight loss. Plus, you'll save tons of time and money by not having to snack all the time. Many people only feel the need to eat twice a day (often skipping breakfast), and some just once a day.

Not having to fight feelings of hunger can also potentially help with problems like sugar or food addiction, and possibly some eating disorders, like bulimia, as well. At least feeling satisfied can be part of the solution. Food can stop being an enemy and become your friend – or simply fuel, whatever you prefer.

Constant energy and mental performance

Ketosis results in a steady flow of fuel (ketones) to the brain, and you avoid big blood sugar swings. This often results in the experience of improved focus and concentration. Any brain fog will be long gone!

A lot of people use keto diets specifically for increased mental performance. Also, many people experience an increase in energy when in ketosis.

On keto, the brain doesn't need carbs. It's fueled 24-7 by ketones, a perfect brain fuel for focus and energy.

Low carb and diabetes reversal Control blood sugar and reverse type 2 diabetes

A keto diet controls blood sugar levels, and is excellent for reversing type 2 diabetes. This has been proven in studies. It makes perfect sense since keto lowers blood-sugar levels and reduces the negative impact of high insulin levels.

As a keto diet may even reverse existing type 2 diabetes, it's likely to be even more effective at preventing it, or reversing pre-diabetes.

Health benefits of Ketogenic Diet

Studies show that Ketogenic diets can help with weight loss and improve health. It can even help fight diabetes, cancer, epilepsy and Alzheimer's.

Keto diet is an effective tool for influencing various diseases of internals and systems:

1.   Heart disease. Keto diet contributes to reducing bad cholesterol, normalization blood pressure and sugar.

2.   Oncological diseases. Keto slows the development of malignant tumors.

3.   Ovaries diseases. The diet reduces the level of insulin, which blocks the formation of cysts on the ovaries.

4.   Skin diseases. Low levels of insulin and bad cholesterol improve the general condition of the skin.

5.   Alzheimer and Parkinson diseases. Ketogenic diet contributes to reducing the symptoms of mental disorders in young and elderly people.

6.   Epileptic disorders. Keto diet leads to a reduction in seizures in children.

CHAPTER 2: COMMON KETOGENIC DIET MISTAKES TO AVOID

It takes a lot of focus and might be a struggle for some since you are completely changing your lifestyle. Your body is making a complete internal change and the way you go about different things in life is going to change too.

There are hundreds of people that switch over to the Keto Dash system and loved it. However, there are many of those people that didn't see some of the results they wanted as fast as they hoped.

Why may you ask?

Because they made some simple, yet common mistakes that many people make when they are on a ketogenic diet.

This is okay. Nobody is perfect and mistakes happen all the time. The important thing to do is learn from your mistakes and understand how you can avoid them from now on.

Common Keto Mistakes

Below is going to be common mistakes that people make on a keto diet. There will also be some tips on how to avoid making these mistakes so you don't make them when you start your journey.

Or, if you've already started your journey, you can learn how to not continue making these mistakes so that you can start seeing the results you want.

Using Keto as a "Quick Fix"

Some people may try to use the keto diet as a quick fix to their body issues.

Ketogenic diets are not a quick fix. It is a lifestyle change that you need to stick with in order to see long-term change.

You may see some changes relatively quickly, but that doesn't mean you can jump right into your old eating habits like before and expect to see those changes stick around. It's very easy to fall back into your old body and you'll be right back to square one.

There are going to be times where you can slip away from the keto diet for a little bit, but you'll be able to slip right back into it quickly once you've tackled it for a while.

Don't think that things are going to be permanently different if you stick with keto for a couple months.

Again, this is a lifestyle change that you need to be prepared to stick with for the long term.

Obsessing Over the Scale

Yes, the diet is designed to help you lose body fat, thus shedding the pounds off your body. However, this is a process and obsessing over your weight is only going to make things harder.

Checking your weight multiple times a day or even on a daily basis is going to make you get in your own head and things will start to slowly go downhill from there.

You have to trust that if you're doing everything the right way, staying away from the sugars and carbs and hitting your macros every day, the weight is going to come off. That's just how it is.

Checking your weight hours apart is going to get you discouraged. You can't expect to see a massive change in weight in a matter of hours. Significant change happens over multiple days and weeks, not hours.

I would suggest that you only check your weight once a week. The same time every week as well. Give yourself a minute time slot on the same day of each week to see the progress you've made up to now. This is when you'll start to actually see the change you're expecting.

Being Afraid of Fats

Most of us growing up were always told that fat is bad for you. Well with this diet, you need to eat fat to lose fat. It sounds like an oxymoron, but it works.

Some people may see that once they've calculated their macros, the amount of fat they have to eat is a massive amount.

On this diet, you may have to consume a large amount of fat to help your body reach the goal you've set for yourself.

About 75% of the food you eat needs to come from fats. That's a high percentage of your food content and may come as a shock to you, but to be successful with this diet, this is how things need to be.

Don't be afraid of the amount of fat you have to eat. Understand that this diet is only going to help you in the end so if you follow everything how it is presented to you, you'll have almost no problems.

Eating the Wrong Fats

To go along with the last mistake, you need to make sure you're eating the right fats.

Don't just assume that since your meeting your daily fats re□uirement that it means you're eating the right kind of fats. There is such a thing as good fats and bad fats.

The bad fats that people may struggle with are the processed fats. This can be found in processed vegetable oils. So, because of this, cooking with these oils is a no-no.

Fats that you want to be consuming are the saturated fats, monounsaturated fats, polyunsaturated fats, and naturally occurring trans fats.

Getting these types of fats are fairly easy when you're looking to avoid all of the processed trans fats.

These good fats can be found in butter, eggs, avocados, walnuts, and fish oils. There are plenty of other sources for these fats, but those are just a few examples.

You can get these fats through fat bombs as well. These are going to give you the fats you may desperately need when you're on this diet.

Adds those to your meals and you'll see that you're hitting your fats requirement while staying with the good fats.

Eating Too Much Protein

To some of you, this may not seem like such a bad thing. You aren't allowed many carbs so a way to supplement that is through consuming protein.

However, having too much protein is going to have negative effects on your body during a keto diet.

Your body only needs so much protein, anything more than that and it starts to get converted into fat. We are trying to eliminate fat so anything that adds fat to your body is a negative.

Avoiding this is pretty simple. All you need to do is focus on your macros. Stay with your macros and you won't have to worry about having anything in excess. You will only have exactly what you need.

Not Enough Water

During a keto diet, your body is going to lose a lot of fluids, so it's important to stay as hydrated as possible. For some reason, people seem to forget about this a lot.

You're losing a lot of fluids and electrolytes that can easily be put back into your body through water.

When you aren't staying hydrated, your body is going to store as much fat as possible. Again, this is the opposite of what we want to happen.

Staying hydrated also means that your organs are going to be working the way they should. Your body will be working like a well-oiled machine.

Some of you may not be used to drinking water constantly throughout the day, but it's something that has to be done. The recommended amount of water is about a gallon a day. Yes, this sounds like a lot, but a few sips here and there throughout the day will make this task a lot more doable.

Besides, if you're going to add in some keto alcohol drinks to your lifestyle you'll need to get as much water in you as possible.

Not Enough Sleep

The process of getting into ketosis, when your body starts using fat as its energy source, can cause you to lose a little bit of sleep. You need to do what you can to get the proper amount of sleep that you need.

Everyone needs sleep and getting the right amount can go a long way.

Not getting the right amount of sleep will prevent your body from functioning as well as it should.

If you're able to get a good nights rest, your body will be better equipped to handle the changes it's starting to go through with the keto diet.

Not Mixing Meals Up

With a keto diet, since you are restricted when it comes to your carb intake, you may think that you are restricted on the number of recipes you can have as well.

Because of this, some people tend to eat the same things all the time.

If you only like certain foods then I can understand this. However, when you start mixing things up, you'll find that the diet is much more enjoyable.

Having a different meal all the time will keep your morale up and allow you to go further with the diet. Make Turkey Pesto Meatballs for one meal then make Grilled Chicken and Spinach White Pizza for the next meal.

Don't forget to add in some low-carb vegetables since not all recipes are going to include vegetables for you to have.

You should always keep your taste buds guessing so some of your favorite foods don't start to become bland if you continue to eat regularly. Nothing is worse than constantly eating your favorite meal, then actually getting sick of it because you've had so often.

Comparing Yourself to Others

This mistake may be the one thing that holds people back more than the others. Simply because it is all mental.

People love comparing themselves to others. It's just a part of human nature. Everyone does it.

When it comes to the keto diet, you cannot compare yourself to others. That is just signing your own death sentence. You need to focus on yourself and nobody else.

Everyone's body is going to react differently to the diet. This means that people are going to experience different weight loss at different rates than you as well.

If anything, when you see somebody's weight loss and it's greater than yours, all you should do is congratulate them and keep encouraging them. Understand that your weight loss is happening and you will reach your goal eventually.

Avoid the Problems

All of these mistakes are easily avoidable. Some of them are physical and some are mental.

The physical mistakes are usually easier to avoid than the mental ones. However, with the kind of supportive community we have at Keto Dash, you should be able to overcome any mental obstacles you may have.

If you happen to make any of these mistakes, just take a step back, re-evaluate how you can stop it from happening again, then get right back at things.

Chapter 3: WHAT TO EAT AND WHAT TO AVOID ON THE KETO DIET

Grocery list for your perfect keto plan

We've covered the nutrient groups you need to intake while you are on a ketogenic diet. The next couple of chapters of the book will deal with the thing that probably interests you the most - what foods to eat during a keto. Before we move on to a suggestion for a diet plan and some of my favorite recipes, let's make a general overview of the foods you should eat and the foods you shouldn't eat while on a ketogenic diet.

Vegetables

Although vegetables are important for a ketogenic diet, you need to make smart choices when it comes to choosing them. The general rule for vegetables is to focus on the leafy green ones.

I will now list the types of vegetables you can freely consume. I suggest you focus on the first several items on the list and limit the intake of root vegetables and nightshades because of their carb amounts:

- Dark, leafy green vegetables – spinach, lettuce, Swiss chard and kale

- Vegetables that have lower carb levels – celery, cucumber, zucchini, squash, asparagus

- Cruciferous vegetables – broccoli, cabbage, Brussels sprouts

- Nightshades – tomatoes, eggplant, and peppers

- Root vegetables – garlic, onion, radishes

- Sea vegetables – Kombu and nori

You might think that all types of vegetables are healthy, but some of them have high carb levels that make them a bad choice for a ketogenic diet. These are:

- Peas, potatoes, corn, parsnips, yucca, yams, beans and legumes

Sauces

The best sauces and other condiments are made from scratch. Pre-made sauces often have added sugars, which aren't a healthy option for your body, especially if you are on a ketogenic diet.

You should think about using a thickener, such as a xanthan gum or guar. It provides a good way to thicken watery sauces and keep them healthy.

Aside from the pre-made sauces, you can use these condiments as long as you read the ingredients:

- Ketchup (no added sugar)

- Mayonnaise (homemade, if possible)

- Mustard

- Hot sauce

- Sauerkraut

- Relish

- Worcestershire sauce

- Horseradish

- Caesar, ranch and other fattier salad dressings

Sweets

Believe it or not, most of the cravings in our organism are caused by sugar. Your cravings can get particularly strong during a ketogenic diet. If you can endure, it is a great idea to restrain from any sweeteners for 30 days. This way you will be able to completely eliminate cravings.

However, this might be a tricky job, so take a look at some sweets that are allowed even if you are on a ketogenic diet:

- Dark chocolate with 70% cocoa is rich in antioxidants

- Inulin — a sweet plant that helps with your blood sugar level

- Stevia, xylitol and similar sweeteners, but don't go for powdered versions but the pure products

Naturally, you should limit the intake of sweets. More important than anything, this is sweet food you should avoid on a keto diet:

- Sugar

- Honey

- High-fructose corn syrup

These have high amounts of sugar and can easily knock you out of ketosis.

Spices

This is a really tricky part as you want to add flavor to your food, but you don't want to make a mistake and significantly increase your intake of carbs.

The important thing when it comes to spices is to read the label because most of the pre-made mixes have added sugar, which is recommended to avoid.

You can safely use :

- Chili powder

- Cayenne pepper

- Oregano

- Cinnamon

- Cumin

- Basil

- Parsley

- Thyme

- Rosemary

- Cilantro

Please note that spices contain carbs and you need to make sure to add them to your calculations.

The good news is that you can freely use salt and pepper as much as you like and there is no need to worry about their nutritional information.

Dairy Products

Dairy provides you with an easy way to add additional fats to your meals. You can be creative and combine them with other food as long as you watch out your protein intake. People who are lactose intolerant should naturally stick to those products that contain less lactose.

The examples of full-fat dairy product you should eat while on a ketogenic diet are:

- Cottage cheese, goat cheese, mozzarella, cheddar and other soft and hard cheeses

- Yogurt

- Sour cream

- Homemade mayonnaise

Remember, it is a much healthier option to choose raw and organic dairy products.

The dairy products you should avoid include:

- Milk – it is high in carbs

- Low-fat products- usually overly processed and stripped of fatty acids and other nutrients

Drinks

Aside from having to eat, you will also have to drink something. In fact, staying hydrated is an important part of every ketogenic diet.

Here are what drinks are allowed :

- Water – your go-to source and the most important way of staying hydrated. Aside from still, you can also drink sparkling water

- Coffee and tea – it improves your concentration, but do not add sugar or milk.

On the other hand, you should make sure not to consume :

- Soft drinks, including diet sodas

- Craft beers and sweet wines, as well as flavored liquor, keep in mind that alcohol slows down the process of losing weight

- Fruit juices

Proteins

There is a wide variety of sources for your protein. The darker meat is a bit fattier than the white meat, but the only rule you should stick to is to be careful not to over-consume on protein. The goal of the ketogenic diet is the state of ketosis, but a higher intake of protein than the one recommended might lower your body's ability to produce ketones and increase the production of glucose.

Here is the list of proteins to eat while you are on keto:

- Meat from pasture-raised or grass-fed animals

- Fish – preferably wild caught, such as catfish, halibut, cod, mackerel, salmon, tuna, trout or snapper

- Shellfish – lobsters, clams, oysters, mussels, scallops, squid

- Organic eggs – they contain a lot of vitamins and fatty acids

The main thing to avoid is eating processed ingredients, which is why you should steer clear of:

- Products from factory-farmed animals and seafood – they are lower in nutrients and more often than not contain preservatives that can cause cancer and affect your health in a negative way

Nuts and Seeds

They a good fat source, but they also have a considerable amount of carbs and proteins, so you need to be careful with the amount you consume. You can use raw nuts to add texture or flavoring to the meals. In general, nuts and seeds should be roasted because that takes away all the anti-nutrients.

These are some nuts and seeds you can consume during keto:

- Macadamia/Brazil nuts, walnuts, pecans, almonds, sunflower and flax seeds

- Flour made from nut and seed is an excellent replacement for regular flour. You can try almond or coconut flour

Aside from limiting the number of nuts and seeds you can consume, you should also avoid:

- Cashews, chestnuts, pistachios, and peanuts because of higher carb levels

Fruits

Fruits usually have a high amount of carbs or sugar and they are not recommended during a ketogenic diet. The only exceptions are avocados and berries, such as blueberries or raspberries, but you should also limit their intake. The same goes for citrus fruit, such as oranges and lemons and their juices (and zest).

Fats

Fats will be the biggest part of your daily calorie intake, so we will start by analyzing them. When you are making choices on which food to eat, always keep in mind your personal taste. The important thing is to select the right types of fats and avoid the wrong ones that disrupt your organism.

There are four fat groups to consider:

- Saturated Fats

- Monounsaturated fats

- Polyunsaturated fats

- Trans fats

You can freely consume saturated and monounsaturated fats, as well as polyunsaturated fats if they are coming from a natural source. Trans fats are the only group of fats you should completely avoid as they have a negative effect on your health.

Here are some suggestions on what you should include in your ketogenic diet:

- Duck fat

- Grass-fed butter

- Tallow

- Ghee

- Egg yolks

- Macadamia

- Olive

- Avocado

- Fish (salmon, trout, tuna, sardines) and animal fat (non-hydrogenated)

- Oils: olive, coconut, macadamia, MCT (choose cold-pressed oils)

Now, here is a list of fats to avoid as they are not healthy for your body:

- Refined oils: canola, sunflower, soybean, corn, grapeseed

- Margarine – even the "heart healthy" one is not good for your health and leads to weight gain and increases stroke risk.

Food List To Avoid On The Keto Diet

Ketogenic foods are high ⬜uality, whole, natural foods processed as little as possible. To avoid processed foods, many keto-ers prefer to make everything themselves, from burgers to homemade ghee).

Ketogenic foods are high in fat, adequate in protein and of course, low carb.

The most common mistakes on a ketogenic diet include not watching the quality and composition of your food and being careless about your carb intake.

To lose weight on keto you must:

- Count carbs — even hidden carbs found in spices, vegetables and drinks.
- Watch your sugar intake: this includes sweeteners, fruit and naturally occurring sugars in dairy. If you must use a sweetener, stick with stevia or opt for other keto-friendly sweeteners.
- Watch your calories. Don't exceed your calorie budget. To lose weight you need to eat less than what you burn. All calculations and metrics are discussed below.
- Be conscious of your food in general. Avoid processed food. No matter how low-carb or "keto" it may be, if it's full of junk you're better off avoiding it.
- Drink plenty of water. Carbs are famous for retaining water, so keto's very low-carb ratio can lead to faster dehydration and constipation. Compensate with water and keto-friendly drinks.
- Try intermittent fasting to avoid late night binges and speed up your ketone production and weight loss.

Chapter 4: KETO FAT BOMBS AND HEALTH BENEFITS

What are fat bombs?

Fat bombs are an original combination of the right ingredients that you can use as delicious snacks, desserts, and main dishes if you are on a keto diet.

They contain more than 85% of fats, they are easy to prepare, and they can have different textures and tastes.

In addition, fat bombs are much more useful than protein products, like meat, fish, and eggs. That is why high protein foods provide the body with an additional protein, which can use only as fuel.

Fat bombs contain many fats and a small number of proteins, so your body can easily burn subcutaneous fat and maintenance of ketosis.

The popularity of fat bombs is incredible. You can use bombs as quick snacks, which provide the body with the necessary energy for several hours.

The basis of fat bombs is coconut oil and milk products with a high-fat content. They contribute to the formation of ketone bodies, which become an important power source.

Fatty bombs have amazing benefits for human health because they include the necessary minerals, vitamins, fat acid (CLA).

Major Advantage of keto fat bombs

1.   Small size. All types of ketogenic bombs differ in their small weight and size because they consist of a fat base.

2.   Healthy fats. As the basis used allow oils and fats, which contain only useful nutrients.

3.   Ease and speed of cooking. You can cook fat bombs due from 5 to 30 minutes.

Health benefits of keto fat bombs

Everyone knows that trans-fats are harmful to the human body. These are by-products of the chemical treatment of hydrogenated oils, which lead to an increase in bad cholesterol and weight gain.

In the opinion of nutritionists, we must receive daily "correct fats", which promote the assimilation of vitamin A, D, E and K. In addition, monounsaturated fats reduce bad cholesterol and support the correct metabolism.

Here are the reasons why you need to cook fat bombs while you are on keto low-carbohydrate diet:

1.　Maintenance of the correct work of a brain.

2.　Improvement of the cardiovascular system and increase in good cholesterol.

3.　Effective weight loss.

4.　Production of quality energy from healthy fats. About 9 calories in one gram. This is more calories than in protein and carbohydrates.

5.　Fast saturation of the body for a long time.

6.　Strengthening of bones and muscles.

7.　Acceleration of transmission of nerve impulses that trigger the process of metabolism.

8.　Digestion of nutrients from other products.

9.　Good flavor and high aesthetic characteristics of fat bombs.

Healthy ingredients for fat bombs

To cook various keto bombs, you can use solid and liquid fat base.

The most popular fat bases are:

- Coconut oil.

- Coconut cream.

- Cream cheese.

- Butter.

Additional fat bases are:

- Animal fat.

- Hard cheese.

- Raw fat bases are:

- Melted butter.

- Nut cheese.

You can receive fat bombs by mixing of various ingredients with a fat base.

Here are the most popular ingredients for the preparation of keto bombs:

- Coconut flakes.

- Nuts.

- Olive oil.

- Seeds.

- Cinnamon.

- Vanilla.

- Cocoa powder.

- Maple syrup.

- Sweetener (sucralose, erythritol).

- Low-sugar berries (bilberry, cowberry, blackberry).

- Low-carb vegetables.

- Bacon.

- Eggs.

- Meat.

- Milk products: butter, cream, yogurt.

- Cheese products: mozzarella, goat cheese, cheddar, parmesan.

- Seeds and nuts: walnuts, almonds, pumpkin seeds, and flax seeds.

- Natural oils: from avocado, olives, and coconut.

- Avocado.

- Low-carb vegetables and greens.

- Spices, herbs, and salt.

- Cheese.

- Sour cream.

- Lemon juice.

- Culinary herbs.

List of useful products that can be included in the keto diet:

- Fat fish: trout, mackerel, tuna, salmon.

- Meat: red meat, white poultry meat, sausages (ham, bacon).

- Eggs.

How to make easy fat bombs?

To make keto fat bombs is quite simple, so even you are a beginner, and you can do it. The process of making bombs consists of four stages:

Step 1 – Choosing the right texture and taste

You need to decide what type of fat bombs you will cook. What it has to be? Sweet, bitter, sour, savory or spicy bombs? Hard, soft or liquid texture? Small or large form?

Step 2 – Choosing the right fat base

You can use the fat base, which will harden or remain soft during cook keto bombs. Coconut oil and butter are the most popular fat bases. If you wish, you can use any of the basics listed in this book.

Vegetarians prefer raw natural bases and meat eaters choose animal fats.

Step 3 – Choosing of additional ketogenic ingredients

After choosing a fat base, proceed to make a keto bomb. Choose additional ingredients from the allowed list of products. Add salt, spices, and herbs to taste.

Step 4 – Compound of all ingredients

When you choose the fat base and additional ingredients, you need to combine all of it into a homogeneous mass, giving it the necessary form. It can be a ball, a round or square bar, a roll or a cupcake.

You must soften fat base, form keto bombs by manually, place in a suitable container (cake forms, food container, tray or plate) and cool in refrigerator.

Equipment and accessories for cooking of keto bombs:

• Silicone molds for cupcakes of various sizes and configurations. They must be made of the food silicone, which withstands the temperature from -40 to +450 degrees.

• Food processor, blender, and manual mixer.

• Microwave oven and heat oven.

• Silicone paddle.

• Sharp knife for cutting

Measurement chart

There are some of the common measurements that you will encounter in this book. It is good you get used to them now

- Dash = 1/8 teaspoon or less

- 3 teaspoons = 1 tablespoon

- 2 tablespoons = 1/8 cup

- 4 tablespoons = ¼ cup

- 5 tablespoons + 1 teaspoon= 1/3 cup

- 8 tablespoons = ½ cup

- 16 tablespoons = 1 cup

- 1 fluid ounce = 2 tablespoons liquid

- 8 fluid ounces = 1 cup

- 2 cup = 1 pint

- 2 pints = 1 quart

- 4 quarts = 1 gallon

- 15 ounces = 1 pound

Chapter 5: SAVORY FAT BOMS RECIPES

Low-carb bombs from cauliflower and parmesan

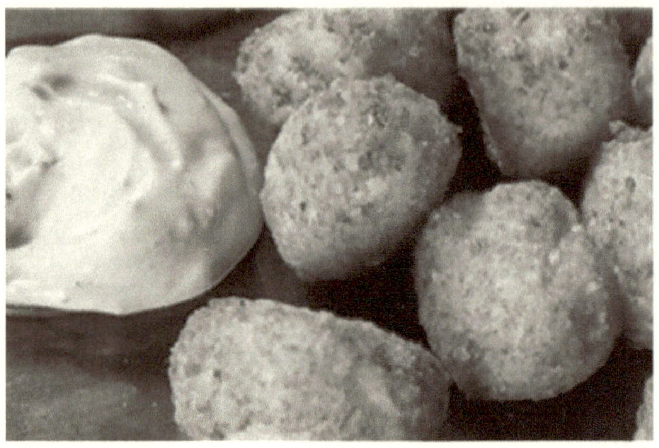

Servings 6-8

Total Time: 30 minutes

Ingredients:

- 1 head cauliflower

- 50 g green onion

- 100 g parmesan

- 100 g Monterey Jack cheese

- 1 egg

- Black ground pepper and salt to taste

- 3 tbsp olive oil

- 2 tbsp mayonnaise

Cooking process:

1.   Cut cauliflower on inflorescences, and grind in a blender until uniformity.

2.   Chop the green onion, and grate the cheese on a fine grater.

3.   In a bowl, mix the cauliflower puree, onion, cheese, and egg. Add salt and pepper to taste. Leave for 20 minutes.

4.   Heat the oil in a deep frying pan. Form the balls by spoon and fry until golden color. Put on paper towels to remove excess fat.

5.   Serve with mayonnaise sauce.

Nutrients per one serving:

Calories: 231 | Fats: 19 g. | Carbohydrates: 3 g. | Proteins: 10 g.

Muffins from cauliflower green chili peppers

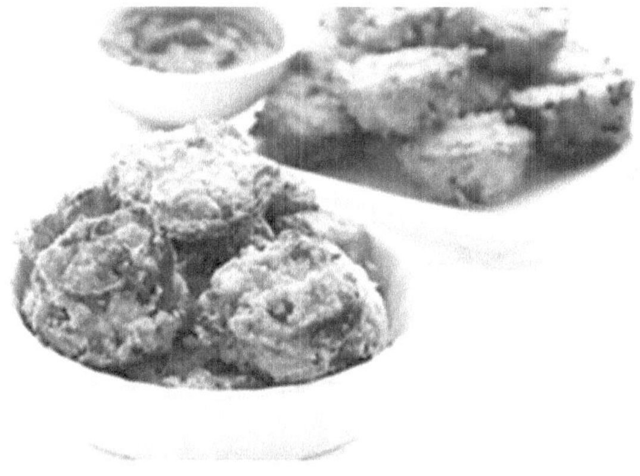

Servings 20

Total Time: 55 minutes

Ingredients:

*   1 head cauliflower

*   100 g cheddar

- ¾ cups almond flour

- 8 slices of bacon

- 1 tbsp dried green chili pepper

- 2 tbsp chopped jalapenos

- 2 eggs

- 2 garlic cloves

- ½ tsp salt

Cooking process:

1.   Cut cabbage on the inflorescence, and blanch of 7 minutes. Grind in a blender until uniformity. Cut bacon into cubes, grate cheese, and chop garlic.

2.   Preheat the oven to 220 °C. To grease the muffins molds.

3.   In a bowl, mix the puree from cauliflower, cheddar, almond flour, bacon, chili, jalapeno, eggs, garlic, and salt. Stir it all thoroughly.

4.   Put the mass into the muffin molds and bake in the oven for 25 minutes until golden color. To cool muffins in a refrigerator before serving.

Nutrients per one serving:

Calories: 205 | Fats: 13.6 g. | Carbohydrates: 8.1 g. | Proteins: 11.5 g.

Keto bombs with cauliflower and bacon

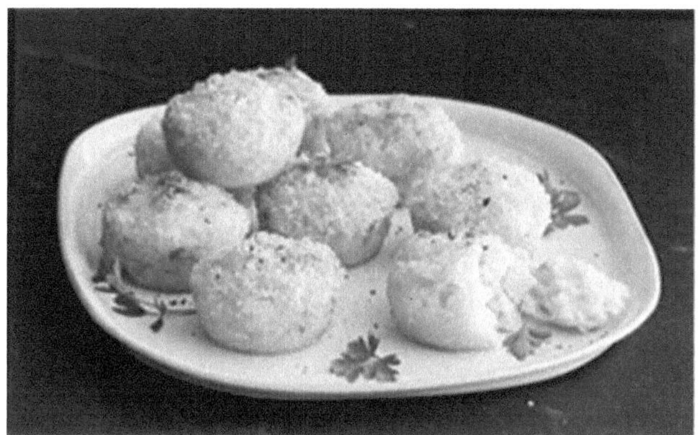

Servings 20

Total Time: 30 minutes + 1 hour for cooling

Ingredients:

- 1 head cauliflower

- 500 g bacon

- 225 g cream cheese

- 120 g goat cheese

- 100 g parmesan

- 100 g cheddar

- 3 garlic cloves

- ½ cup breadcrumbs

- 1 tsp Italian spices

- 1 tsp onion powder

- 1 tsp garlic powder

- ½ tsp sea salt

- ¼ tsp ground black pepper

- 3 tbsp olive oil

Cooking process:

1. Divide the cabbage on inflorescences, and blanch for 5 minutes. Put the cabbage in a blender, and beat to uniformity.

2. Cut bacon into small cubes, and fry it in a dry frying pan for 5 minutes. Grind cream cheese, grate cheddar and parmesan and chop goat cheese.

3. In a deep bowl, mix the cabbage, bacon, goat cheese, cream cheese, and cheddar, chopped garlic, Italian spices, black pepper, and salt. Mix all ingredients thoroughly and refrigerate for 1 hour.

4. In a bowl, mix parmesan, breadcrumbs, garlic and onion powder. You can use this mix as a breading.

5. Form balls with a diameter of 5 cm from cabbage mass and roll them in breadcrumbs.

6. Heat the oil on a deep frying pan. Fry the bombs in hot oil until golden color. Cool them.

Nutrients per one serving:

Calories: 281 | Fats: 19 g. | Carbohydrates: 5.5 g. | Proteins: 18 g.

Cheese muffins with bacon

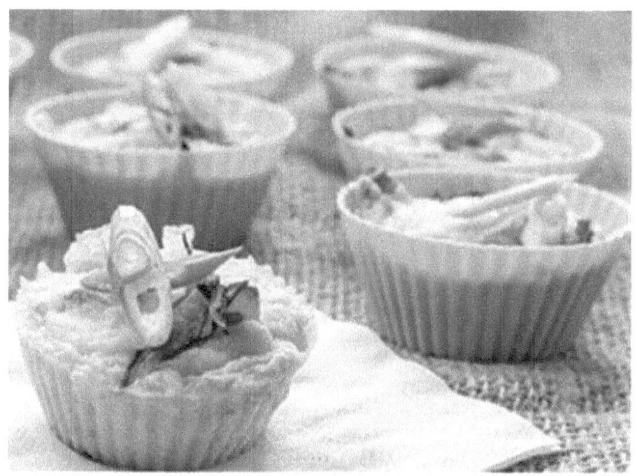

Servings 10

Total Time: 30 minutes

Ingredients:

- 10 slices of bacon

- 50 g green onion

- 5 eggs

- ¼ tsp salt

- ½ tsp ground black pepper

- 100 g cheddar

Cooking process:

1. Grate the cheese, cut bacon into small cubes, and chop the green onion.

2. Heat the oven to 190 °C.

3. Fry the bacon in a dry frying pan for 5 minutes. Add green onion, stir and fry for 2 minutes. Cool the bacon.

4.   In a bowl, break the eggs, add salt and pepper, whisk until uniformity. If desired, you can use a submersible blender.

5.   Pour for 2 tablespoons of egg mass into each form for muffins. Distribute the fried bacon and pour the remaining egg.

6.   Lay out for 1 tablespoon of grated cheese from above. Bake in the oven for 10 minutes. Cool down muffins.

Nutrients per one serving:

Calories: 180 | Fats: 15 g. | Carbohydrates: 0 g. | Proteins: 9 g.

Spicy keto cheese bombs

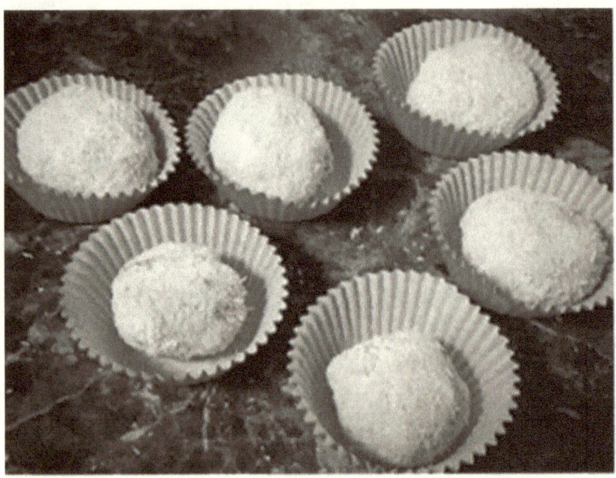

Servings 6

Total Time: 35 minutes

Ingredients:

*   100 g cream cheese

*   60 g butter

*   1 tsp dried basil

*   1 tsp dried thyme

- 1 tsp dried oregano

- 5 dried tomatoes

- 5 pitted olives

- 2 garlic cloves

- ¼ tsp salt

- 30 g parmesan

Cooking process:

1. Cut the butter into small pieces and add to the cream cheese. Mix until uniformity.

2. Add crushed dried tomatoes, olives, and dried greens. Season with salt to taste. Stir and cool them for 20 minutes.

3. Form six balls from the cooled cheese mass. Roll each ball in a grated parmesan.

Nutrients per one serving:

Calories: 163 | Fats: 17.1 g. | Carbohydrates: 1.7 g. | Proteins: 3.7 g.

Keto fat bombs with bacon

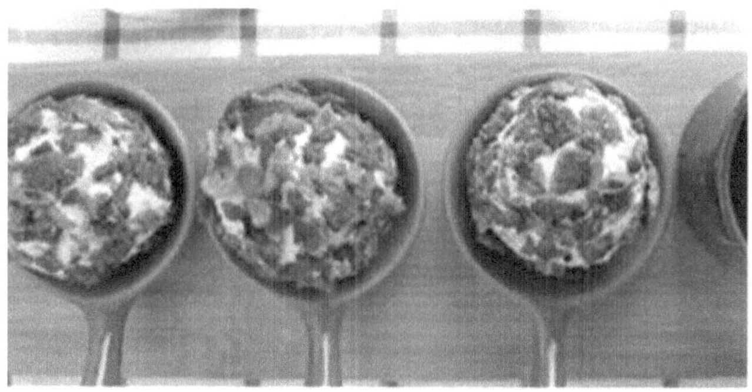

Servings 6-8

Total Time: 25 minutes

Ingredients:

- 100 g butter

- 2 eggs

- 100 g coconut milk

- 100 g bacon

- 3 tbsp coconut flour

- 1 tbsp stevia

- ¼ tsp salt

Cooking process:

1. Heat the oven to 190 °C.

2. Melt the butter in a saucepan. Chop the bacon. In a bowl, mix coconut milk, eggs, coconut flour, salt, and stevia. Add melted butter and chopped bacon to mass. Mix it all.

3. Pour the mass into silicone molds for cupcakes. Bake bombs in the oven for 15 minutes. Put out from an oven, and cool down them.

Nutrients per one serving:

Calories: 150 | Fats: 8.1 g. | Carbohydrates: 5.6 g. | Proteins: 1.6 g.

Bacon Cheeseburger Bombs

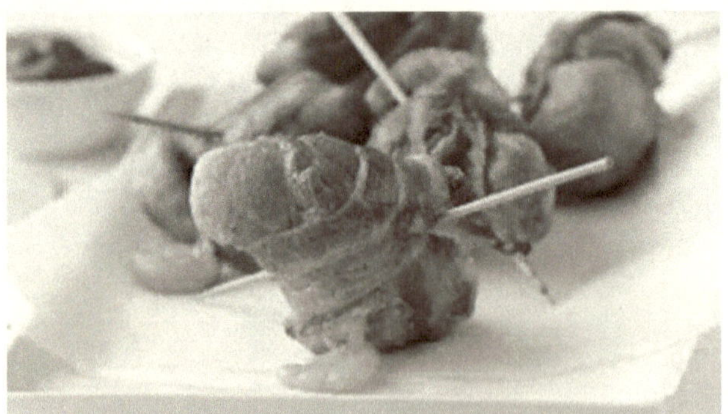

Serving: 10 people

Prep Time: 20 min

Ingredients

* 1 can of Pillsbury Biscuits (10 biscuits)

* 1 pound of lean ground beef

* ½ finely chopped onion

* 2 tablespoons of barbecue sauce

* 1 teaspoon of yellow mustard

* 1 teaspoon Worcestershire sauce

* 5 oz. of cheddar cheese

* 1 egg white

* Sesame seeds

* 3 slices of chopped bacon

* ⅓ Cup of cream cheese

* 1 tablespoon of ketchup

Instructions

* Preheat the oven up to 375 degrees.

* In some large pan, brown bacon, ground beef and the onion until well cooked, then drain any grease.

* Add cream ketchup, barbecue sauce, cheese, mustard, and the Worcestershire sauce.

* Stir over low heat until the cream cheese melts. Allow these to cool.

* Roll every biscuit very thin. Put 2 tablespoons of beef mixture on every biscuit then add 1 square cheese. Wrap your biscuit round

beef/cheese then tightly seal edges.

•   Put your biscuits on a pan lined with parchment then seam side down. Brush using egg white then sprinkle with the sesame seeds.

•   Place them in an oven then turn down heat up to 350 degrees.

•   You can then bake for 13-16 minutes or till lightly browned.

•   Serve when warm.

Nutrients per one serving: Total carbs 2.3g, Fiber 06g, Protein 3.6g, Fat 34.6g, Magnesium 15mg, Potassium 94mg

Cheesy Jalapeno

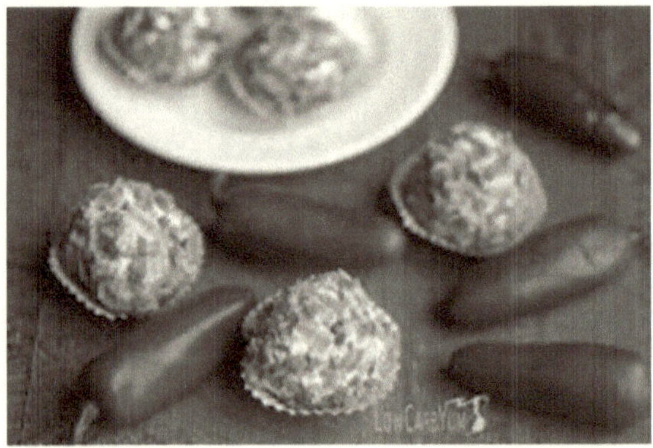

Serving: 2 people

Prep Time: 10 min

Cook Time 30 min

Ingredients

•   4 slices of bacon

•   1/4 cup of grated Gruyère cheese or a Cheddar cheese

•   1/4 cup of unsalted butter or a ghee at room temperature

•   3.5 ounces of full-fat cream cheese

- 2 g jalapeño of finely chopped peppers halved and seeded

Instructions

- In some bowl, mash together cream cheese and the butter or ghee, or just process in your food processor until they are smooth.

- Preheat oven up to 325°F.

- Line rimmed baking sheet with a parchment paper.

- Lay bacon slices flat on parchment

- Place your sheet in preheated oven then cook for about 25 to 30 minutes.

- Remove from oven and set aside to cool. Once cool, crumble bacon into the bowl then set aside.

- To cream cheese and the butter mixture, just add Gruyère or the Cheddar cheese, the jalapeños, and the bacon grease then mix well so as to combine. Refrigerate for about 1 hour.

- Divide your mixture into some 6 fat bombs then place them on a parchment-lined plate.

Nutrients per one serving: Calories 142, Total Fat 15g, Total Carbs 0.9g, Protein 3.5g

Bacon Herb Cream Cheese

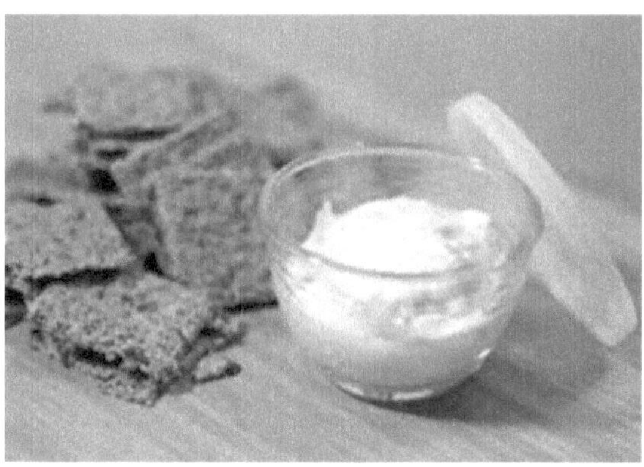

Serving: 2 people

Prep Time: 30 min

Ingredients

- 1/2 cup of Parmesan cheese, grated

- 1/4 cup of bacon bits

- 1 cup of kefir cream cheese/yogurt cream cheese

- 2 cloves of garlic

- 1 tsp of fresh oregano, chopped

- Salt and fresh cracked pepper

- 1/2 cup of bacon fat, room temperature

Instructions

- Add cream cheese to your food processor. Run processor so as to loosen up cream cheese.

- Add the garlic cloves and salt and pepper then run your food processor.

- Pour some thin stream of the liquid bacon fat solely through a hole in the top of a food processor, until well fully incorporated.

- Place contents of food processor into the bowl.

- Add remaining ingredients then fold into mixture. Divide this into 6 smaller portions then refrigerate.

Nutrients per one serving: 89 Calories, 10g Fat, trace g Protein, 1g Carbohydrate, trace g Dietary Fiber, 1g Effective Carbs

Buttered Bacon

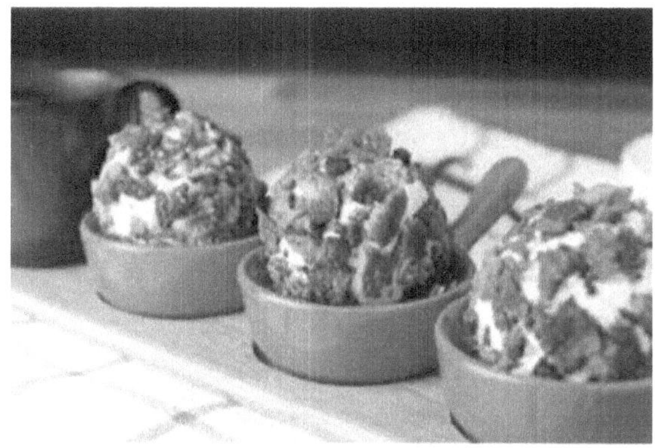

Serving: 3 fat bombs

Prep Time: 2 min

Total Time: 2 min

Ingredients

- 2 toasted & chopped pecan halves

- 1/16 serving of Keto Craisin

- 1 bacon slice

- 1 tablespoon of unsalted Kerrygold butter

Instructions

• Divide the bacon into 3 parts. Slather each part with 1 teaspoon Kerrygold unsalted butter.

• Press the butter side into the pecan pieces. Top each with some Keto Craisin, then repeat until you have eaten all the bacon.

Nutrients per one serving: 158 Calories; 2g Protein, 17g Fat, 1g Carbohydrate, 1g Effective Carbs, trace Dietary Fiber

Butter Pecan

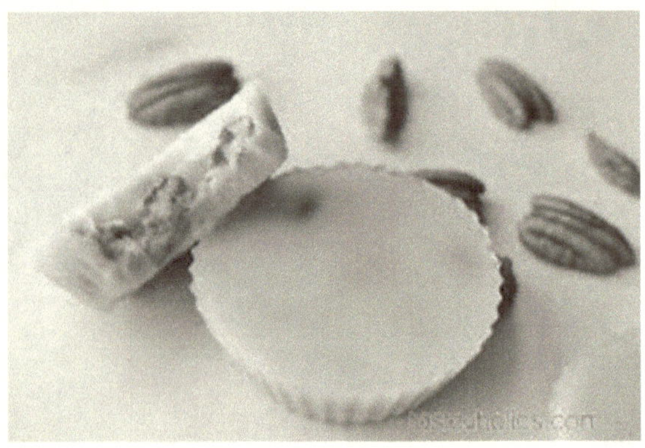

Serving: 2 fat bombs

Prep Time: 1 min

Total Time: 1 min

Ingredients

*   1/2 tablespoon of grass-fed butter, unsalted

*   4 pecan of halves, toasted

*   1 pinch of sea salt

Instructions

*   Spread half of grass-fed butter between the two pecan halves. Use some tiny bit of the sea salt then boom!

Nutrients per one serving: 89 Calories, 10g Fat, 1g Carbohydrate, trace g Protein, 1g Effective Carbs, trace g Dietary Fiber

Zucchini fat bombs

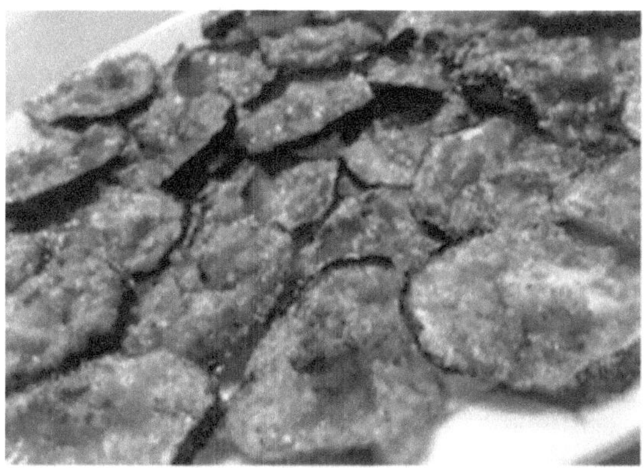

Servings 8

Total Time: 15 minutes + 1 hour for freezing

Ingredients:

* 2 zucchini

* 2 tbsp coconut oil

* 3 tbsp gelatin

* 2 tsp lemon juice

* ¼ tsp sea salt

* 1 tbsp chopped fresh parsley

* 1 tbsp chopped fresh basil

Cooking process:

1.   Cut the zucchini into small cubes, and simmer for 5 minutes.

2.   Cover the baking sheet with parchment.

3.   Mix the zucchini with coconut oil and lemon juice, beat in a blender until uniformity for 1 minute.

4.	Add gelatin and salt to the mass. Beat in a blender next 30 seconds.

5.	Pour the mass into the mold, sprinkle with greens on top. Cool before full hardening. Cut into portions.

Nutrients per one serving:

Calories: 44 | Fats: 3 g. | Carbohydrates: 3 g. | Proteins: 1 g.

Savory Mediterranean

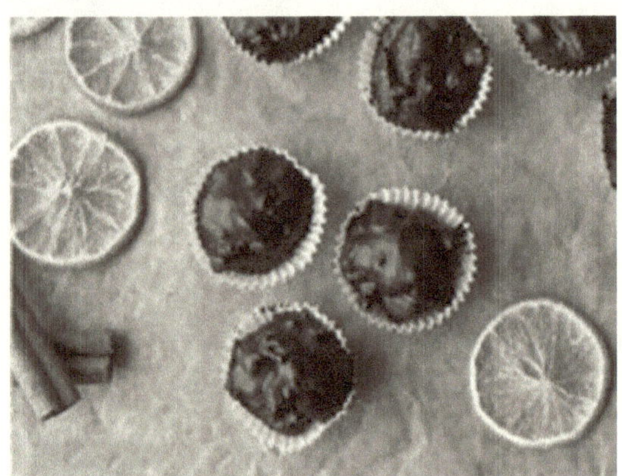

Serving: 6 people

Prep Time: 30 min

Ingredients

*	½ cup of cream cheese, full-fat

*	2 cloves of garlic, crushed

*	Freshly ground black pepper

*	¼ tsp of salt or more to taste

*	¼ cup of softened butter or ghee

*	2-3 tbsps. of freshly chopped herbs

*	4 pieces of drained sun-dried tomatoes

- 4 olives, pitted or kalamata

- 5 tbsps. of grated parmesan cheese

Instructions

- Cut butter into small pieces then place in some bowl with cream cheese. Leave it in the kitchen counter for about 20-30 minutes so as to soften. Mash using a fork then mix until combined. Add in the chopped sun-dried tomatoes as well as the chopped kalamata olives.

- Add the freshly chopped herbs, crushed garlic then seasons using salt and pepper.

- Mix well then place in some fridge for about 20-30 minutes so as to solidify.

- Remove cheese mixture from the fridge then start to create 5 balls. Roll every ball in grated parmesan cheese then place on a plate.

Nutrients per one serving: Total carbs 2g, Fiber 0.3g, Protein 3.7g, Fat 17.1g

Savory Salmon

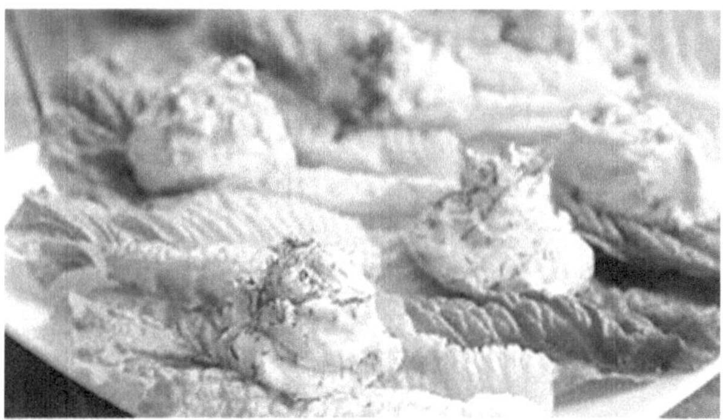

Serving: 6 people

Prep Time: 1 hr. 30 min

Ingredients

*   1 tbsp. of fresh lemon juice

*   1-2 tbsps. of freshly chopped dill

*   Optionally: pinch of salt

*   ½ cup of full-fat cream cheese

*   ⅓ Cup of grass-fed butter

*   ½ package of smoked salmon or a smoked mackerel

Instructions

*   Place butter, cream cheese and smoked salmon into your food processor.

*   Add the fresh lemon juice and the dill then pulse until they are smooth.

*   Line some tray with parchment paper then create small fat bombs by use of 2 ½ tablespoons of your mixture per piece. Garnish using extra dill then place in a fridge for about 1-2 hours or until it becomes firm.

Nutrients per one serving: Total Carbs: 0.8g, Fiber 0.1g, Protein 3.2g, Fat 15.7g

Keto fat snacks from cheese and smoked salmon

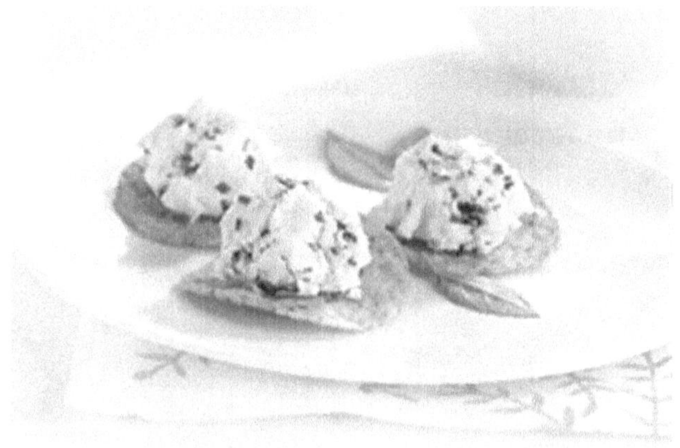

Servings 15

Total Time: 15 minutes

Ingredients:

- 225 g goat cheese

- 1 tbsp fresh rosemary

- 1 tbsp fresh basil

- 1 tbsp oregano

- 2 garlic cloves

- 100 g smoked salmon

- A pinch of salt and black pepper

- Salted crackers or chips

Cooking process:

1.   Cut rosemary, basil, and oregano. Chop garlic. Cut the salmon into small cubes.

2.   In a bowl, mix salmon, goat cheese, herbs, garlic, black pepper, and salt.

3.   Lay out cheese mix by a teaspoon on crackers or chips, and cool for 5 minutes.

Nutrients per one serving:

Calories: 46.2 | Fats: 3.3 g. | Carbohydrates: 0.93 g. | Proteins: 3.4 g.

Keto cheese sauce from a core of coconut palm

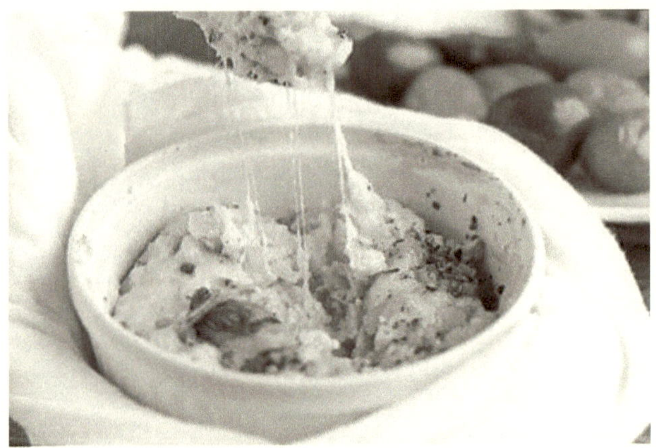

Servings 6-8

Total Time: 30 minutes

Ingredients:

•   1 dry core coconut palm

•   50 g green onion

•   ¼ cup mayonnaise

•   2 tbsp Italian spices

•   100 g parmesan

•   2 eggs

Cooking process:

1.   Preheat the oven to 170 °C. Prepare a form for baking.

2.   Cut the coconut palm core into cubes, chop the onion finely, and grate the cheese on a fine grater.

3.   Lay out the coconut palm core, onion, spices, ½ part of cheese and mayonnaise in a blender, to whisk for 1 minute.

4.   Add one whole egg and yolk to the received mass. To whisk again for 1 minute.

5.   Pour the mass into the form and bake in the oven for 20 minutes. Get out from the oven and sprinkle with the cheese 10 minutes later.

6.   Serve cheese sauce with salt crackers.

Nutrients per one serving:

Calories: 116.1 | Fats: 9.14 g. | Carbohydrates: 2.87 g. | Proteins: 4.93 g.

Peanut Butter Chips

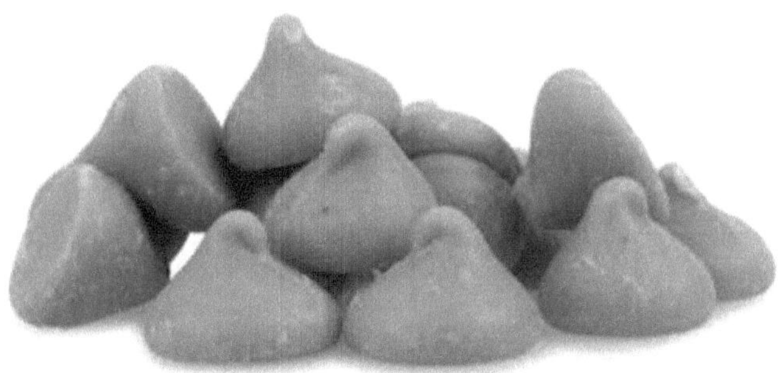

Serving: 2 people

Prep Time 15 min

Total Time 15 min

Ingredients

*   1/4 cups of unsweetened peanut butter powder

- 1/3 cup of Natvia powder

- 100 grams of cocoa butter melted

- 1/2 teaspoon of sea salt

Instructions

- Powder granular sweetener in some NutriBullet type blender or your then set aside.

- Melt the cocoa butter with some sea salt in a chocolate melter, or microwave.

- Stir in the peanut butter powder, the powdered sweetener, and the sea salt until they are well combined.

- Spread the mixture out on the parchment paper, a silicone mat, or a shallow baking pan lined using plastic wrap placed over little water.

- If you need, cover using a parchment paper and smooth out the top with hand.

- Place in a freezer for 30 minutes.

- Remove peanut butter sheet from the pan then cut into small chunks.

Nutrients per one serving: 52 calories, 8mg sodium, 3.7g fat, 3.2g carbs, 1.0g erythritol, 1.1g fiber, 4.4g protein, 1.1g net carbs

Sesame Keto Buns

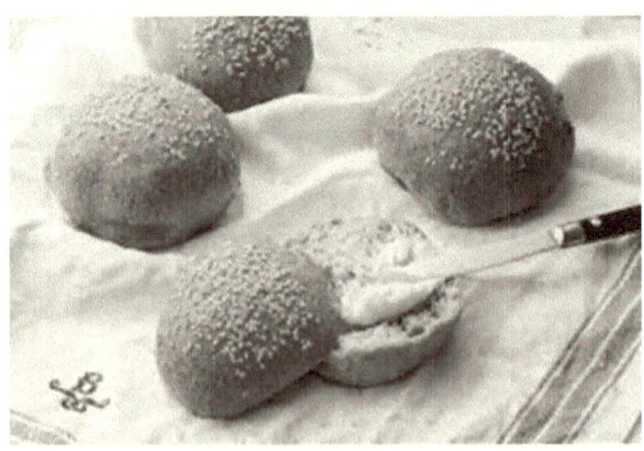

Serving: 12 buns

Prep time: 15 min

Cook time: 50 min

Ingredients

- ½ cup of psyllium powder

- 1 cup of hot water

- ½ cup of sesame seeds and ½ cup for covering the buns

- ½ cup of pumpkin seeds

- 1 tbs of baking powder

- 1 tbs of Celtic sea salt

- 1 cup of coconut flour

- 8 egg whites

Instructions

- Pre-heat your oven up to 350 degrees.

- Combine all the dry ingredients in the large bowl.

- Mix well.

- In some blender, blend egg whites until they are very foamy.

- Add foamy egg whites to dry ingredients then mix well using a spoon, or in a food processor.

- The dough will still be crumbly.

- Add 1 cup of the boiling water to mix then keep stirring until the smoother dough forms.

- The dough will remain to be crumbly but it will stick when formed into a bun.

- Press the buns into the plate where the ½ cup of the sesame seeds was poured, so seeds will stick to the top.

- Place some sheet of the parchment paper on the cookie sheet.

- Place the buns on paper.

- Bake for 50 minutes at 350

- Let cool inside oven for an extra crunchy top.

- Serving 12 small buns

Nutrients per one serving: Calories 133, Fat 6.5g, Fiber 9.5g, Protein 6.9g

Beef Machaca Keto Muffins

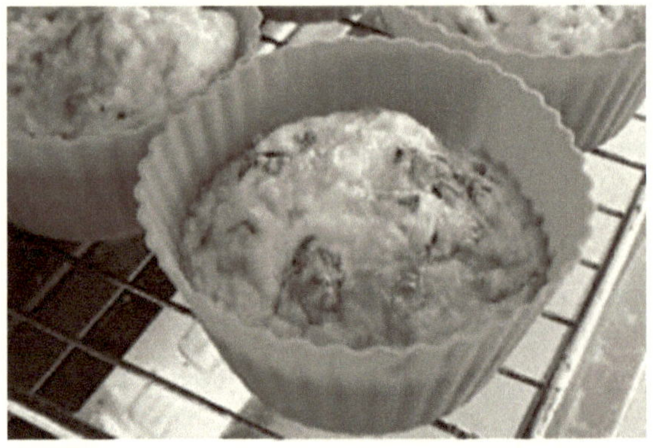

Serving: 8 muffins

Prep time: 10 min

Cook time: 30 min

Ingredients

- 2 tablespoons steak drippings, or the bacon drippings

- ½ cup of Beef Jerky Machaca

- 4 organic eggs

- ½ cup of roasted tomatillo salsa

- ½ cup of almond flour

Instructions

- Pre-heat the oven up to 350 degrees.

- In your 7" nonstick ceramic pan placed on a medium heat, just melt fat of choice then add machaca to it.

- Stir for 3 minutes or for the machaca to soften and fragrant.

- Allow cooling for about 5 minutes.

- In a food processor, just add eggs, almond flour, tomatillo salsa, and machaca.

- Mix on low for 30 seconds, or until all the ingredients become well blended.

- Pour the mixture into some 8 silicone muffin cups, or into silicone muffin mold.

- Bake for 30 minutes at 350 degrees or until the toothpick becomes clean when it has been inserted into the muffin.

Nutrients per one serving: Calories 128, Fat 10g, Fiber 0.75g, Protein 6.6g

Baked Pecan Prosciutto and Brie Savory

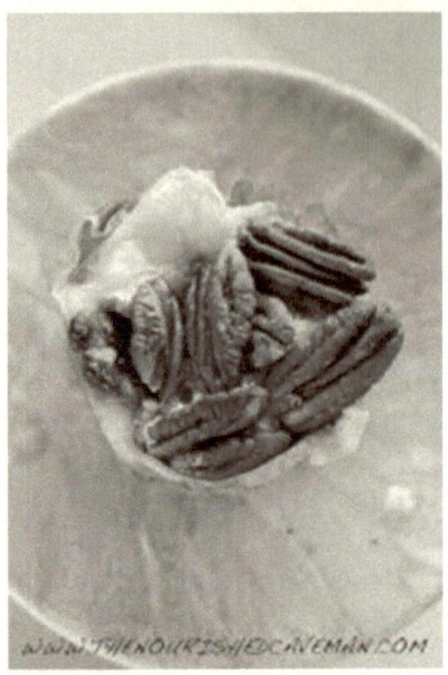

Serving: 1 serving

Prep time: 5 min

Cook time: 12 min

Ingredients

*   6 pecan halves

*   ⅛ Teaspoon of black pepper

*   1 slice of prosciutto

*   1 ounce of full-fat Brie cheese

Instructions

*   Preheat the oven up to 350°F.

*   Take a slice of prosciutto then fold it into half to become almost square.

*   Place it in the hole of the muffin tin so as to line it up completely.

- • Chop Brie into little cubes, while leaving the white skin on. Put Brie in the prosciutto-lined cup.

- • Stick pecan halves in the Brie.

- • Bake for 12 minutes, until the Brie becomes melted and the prosciutto is cooked.

- • Cool for about 10 minutes before you can remove from muffin pan.

Nutrients per one serving: Calories 183, Fats 16.50g, Fiber 1g, Protein 8.42g

Maple & Pecan Fudge

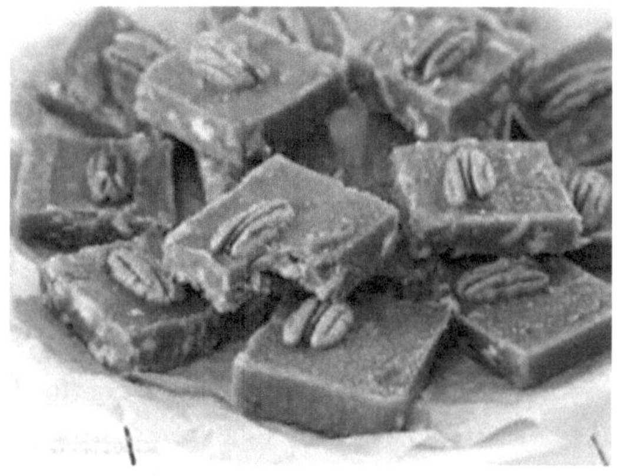

Serving: 16 people

Prep Time: 2 hours

Ingredients

Spiced Maple & Pecan Butter:

- • ½ tsp of vanilla powder or 1 tsp of vanilla extract

- • 1 tsp of sugar-free maple extract

- • 3 cups of pecans or walnuts

- • Pinch salt

Maple & Pecan Fudge:

- ½ cup of unsalted butter or a coconut oil

- 1 ¼ cup of chopped pecans plus 16 pecan halves

1 recipe of Maple & Pecan Butter

- ¼ cup of powdered Erythritol or a Swerve

- 10-20 drops of liquid stevia

Instructions

- Start by making Spiced Maple and Pecan Butter. In your food processor, combine pecans, vanilla, maple extract, cinnamon, and salt.

- Process until they are smooth for some few minutes. Use a spatula to scrape your mixture from sides if needed.

- Add the Erythritol and the butter.

- Pulse until smooth.

- Transfer your dough to 8 x 8-inch parchment-lined pan, or some silicone pan. By use of a spatula, spread dough evenly into pan.

- Add some roughly chopped pecans then mix in.

- Top with the rest of pecan halves. Refrigerate them for about 1 to 2 hours.

- Be sure your fudge has been set before you can slice. Keep refrigerated for about 1 week or just freeze for about 3 months.

Nutrients per one serving: Total Carbs 4.2g, Fiber 2.8g, Protein 2.6g, Fat 26g

Cookie Dough

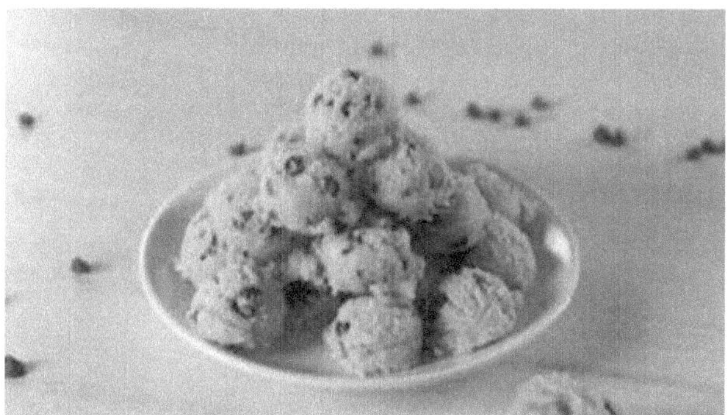

Serving: 10 people

Prep Time: 5 min

Ingredients

- 1 tablespoon of maple syrup or some 10 drops of liquid stevia

- 1/4 cup of almond Yum butter or the almond butter

- 1/4 cup of dark chocolate, finely chopped

- 3/4 cup of almond flour

- 1/2 cup of coconut oil, melted

Instructions

- In some bowl, combine almond butter, coconut oil, maple syrup, almond flour then mix well.

- Fold in the chocolate.

- Transfer to loaf pan then freezes until set.

- Cut into squares then store in an airtight container kept in the fridge.

Nutrients per one serving: Calories: 209, Fat: 19.9 g, Unsaturated fat: 9g, Saturated fat: 10.9 g, Trans fat: 0 g, Sugar: 3.7 g, Carbohydrates: 6.7 g, Sodium: 4 mg Fiber: 1.3 g, Cholesterol: 1 mg, Protein: 3.4 g

Savory Pizza

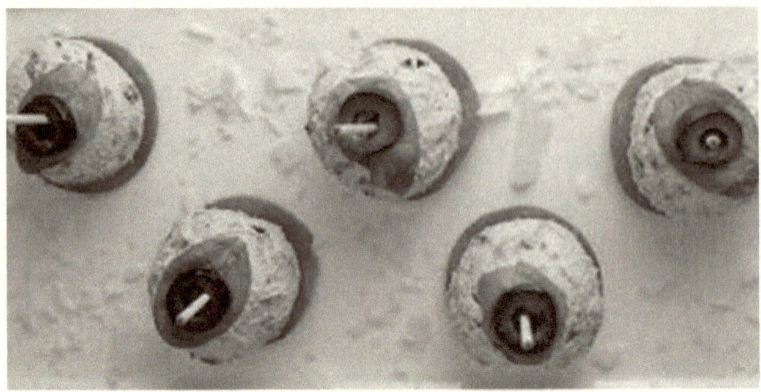

Serving: 4 people

Prep Time: 1 hr. 30 min

Ingredients

- 2 tbsp. of Sun-Dried Tomato Pesto

- 2 tbsp. of Fresh Basil, chopped

- 4 oz. of Cream Cheese

- 14 slices of Pepperoni

- 8 pitted of Black Olives

- Salt and Pepper

Instructions

- Dice the pepperoni and the olives into some small pieces.

- Mix together the basil, tomato pesto, and the cream cheese.

- Add the olives and the pepperoni into cream cheese then mix again.

- Form into balls, and garnish with basil, pepperoni, and olive.

Nutrients per one serving: 110 Calories, 1.3g Net Carbs, 10.5g Fats, and

2.3g Protein.

Breakfast Bacon

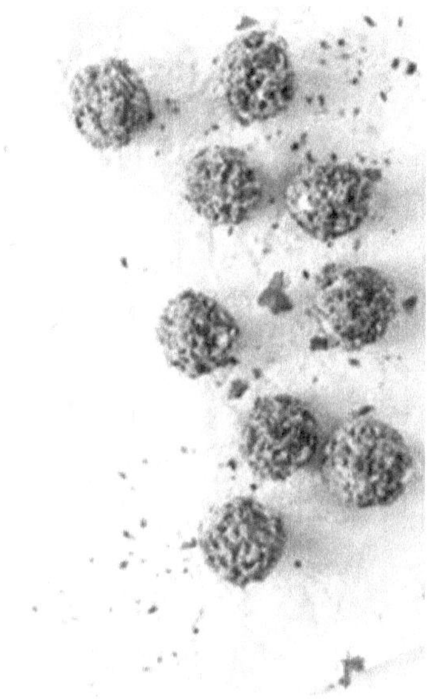

Serving: 6 people

Prep time: 30 min

Cook Time: 20 min

Ingredients

- 1 Large Hardboiled Egg

- ¼ Avocado

- 4 tbsps. of Unsalted or Clarified Butter

- 1 tbsp. of Mayonnaise

- 1 seeded and diced Serrano Pepper

- 1 tbsp. of Cilantro, chopped

- Kosher Salt

- Cracked Pepper

- Juice of ¼ Lime

- 2 tbsps. of Bacon Grease

- 6 Bacon Slices, Cooked

Instructions

- In some large bowl, combine avocado, butter, hardboiled egg, mayonnaise cilantro, and serrano pepper. Mash into a smooth paste using a fork or a potato masher. Season using salt and pepper, and add lime juice and stir.

- Prepare the bacon in favorite fashion until it becomes crispy while reserving 2 tablespoons bacon grease. Add bacon grease to fat bomb mixture then stir gently. Cover then place in a fridge for about 30 minutes, or until your mixture is cooled and can be formed into solid balls. Crumble bacon into some small bits in some small bowl.

- Use a spoon to scoop out 6 amounts of fat bomb mixture then form into balls. Just add balls to bacon bits then roll around until they are completely covered.

- Serve immediately.

Nutrients per one serving: Calories: 103, Fat: 9g, Carbohydrates: 1g, Fiber: 0g, Protein: 7g

Bacon Wrapped Mozzarella Sticks

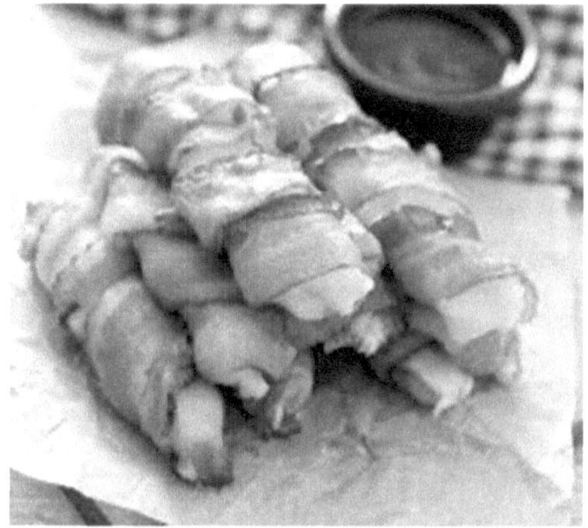

Serving: 2 people

Prep time: 10 min

Cook time: 3 min

Ingredients

- 1 Frigo of cheese heads cheese stick, mozzarella

- 2 slices bacon

- Coconut oil

- Low sugar pizza sauce(optional)

- Toothpicks

Instructions

- Preheat the coconut oil in deep fryer up to 350 degrees.

- Wrap your cut into half cheese sticks and bacon, while overlapping them.

- Drop the bacon already wrapped with cheese in hot oil then cook until bacon becomes quite brown.

- Remove to the paper towel so as to cool for a few minutes. Remove toothpick then enjoy with favorite dipping sauce!

Nutrients per one serving: Calories: 103, Fat: 9g, Carbohydrates: 1g, Fiber: 0g, Protein: 7g

Cheese, Jalapeno and Bacon Bite

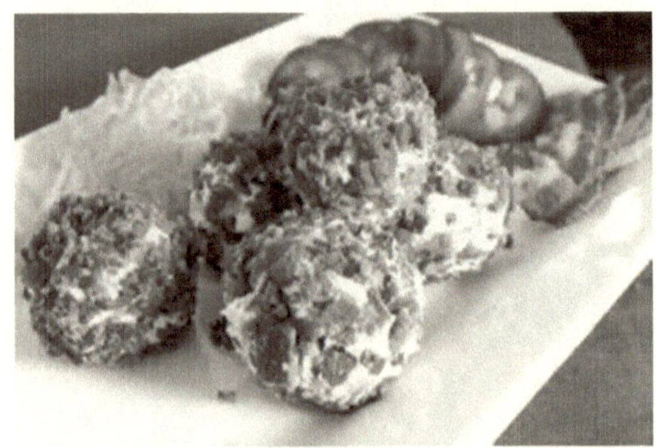

Serving: 20 people

Prep Time: 20 min

Cook Time: 20 min

Ingredients

- 4 jalapeno peppers

- 3 ounces of coconut oil, expeller-pressed

- 2 ounces of bacon grease

- 8 ounces of full-fat cream cheese or the dripped yogurt cheese

- 4 slices of chopped and cooked bacon, grease reserved

- 4 ounces of shredded cheddar cheese

Instructions

- Melt coconut oil in case it is solid.

- Cook the bacon over medium heat and in a medium skillet.

- Dice the Jalapeno peppers after removal of stems then rinsing out the seeds.

- Combine the cheddar cheese, cream cheese, bacon grease, diced Jalapeno, and melted coconut oil.

- Press the cream cheese mixture to parchment-lined loaf pan then chill for about 2-3 hours.

- Set the bacon pieces aside.

- Once the cream cheese mixture has become firm, remove from the loaf pan then cut into 18 pieces.

- Gently roll them into balls then roll the balls into the crumbled bacon as you desire.

- Enjoy immediately or keep before you can cover in the bacon in a fridge for about 5 days or in a freezer for about 4 weeks.

Nutrients per one serving: Calories 134, Saturated fat. 9 g, Fat 13 g, Trans fat: 0 g, Sugar: 1 g, Sodium: 107 mg, Carbohydrates: 1 g, Fiber: 0 g, Protein: 3 g

Cream cheese appetizer with bacon

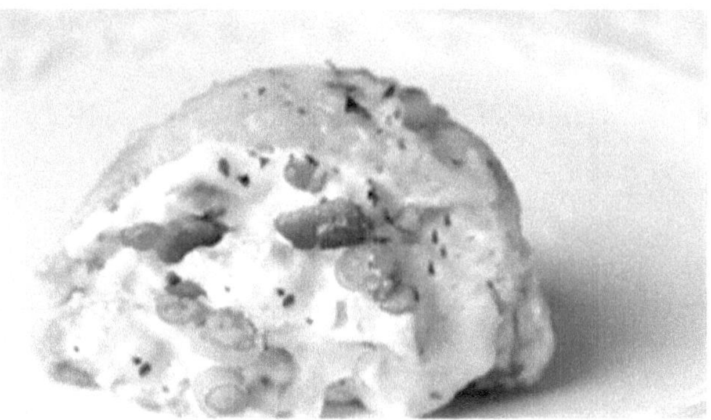

Servings 8

Total Time: 25 minutes

Ingredients:

- 225 g cream cheese

- 225 g bacon

- 50 g green onion

- 50 g parmesan

- 50 g cheddar

- 1 tsp garlic powder

- 200 g biscuit cookies

Cooking process:

1.   In a bowl, mix cream cheese, chopped bacon, onion, garlic powder, grated parmesan, and salt.

2.   Lay out the biscuit on a baking sheet covered with parchment. Lay out the cream mass by a tablespoon on the cookies. Sprinkle with grated cheddar cheese.

3.   Bake in the oven for 15 minutes at a temperature of 190 °C.

Nutrients per one serving:

Calories: 453 | Fats: 32 g. | Carbohydrates: 30 g. | Proteins: 10 g.

Keto cheese appetizer with broccoli

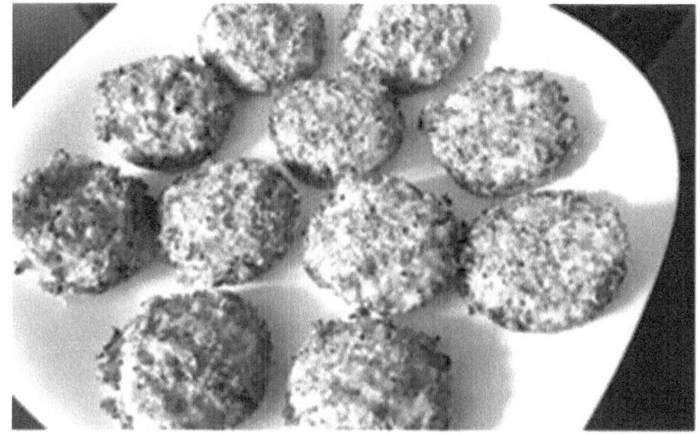

Servings 12

Total Time: 40 minutes

Ingredients:

- 1 head of broccoli

- 200 g cheddar cheese

- 2 eggs

- ¼ tsp Himalayan salt

- ¼ tsp ground black pepper

- 1 tbsp butter

Cooking process:

1. Cut the broccoli into the inflorescence. Lay out into a blender and grind until uniformity. Grate cheddar on a fine grater.

2. In a deep bowl, mix broccoli, grated cheddar, eggs, pepper, and salt.

3. Preheat the oven to 200 degrees.

4. Grease muffin molds. Lay out a mix into molds and gently level it.

5.   Bake in the oven for 30 minutes until golden color. Cool the appetizer and lay out on a dish.

Nutrients per one serving:

Calories: 83 | Fats: 6 g. | Carbohydrates: 0.9 g. | Proteins: 5.8 g.

Flourless Paleo Keto Bomb

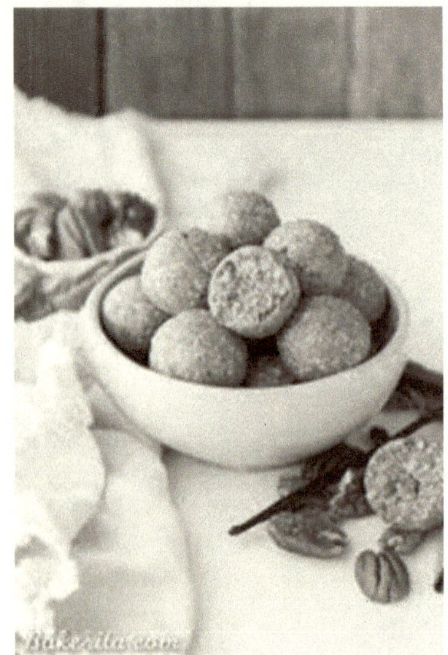

Serving: 16 people

Prep Time 10 min

Cook Time 25 min

Ingredients

- 1 1/4 teaspoon of monk fruit liquid extract

- 2 teaspoons of vanilla extract

- 1/4 cup of unsweetened cocoa

- 1/2 cup of coconut oil

- 8 ounces of unsweetened baking chocolate

- 3 large eggs or some 2 duck eggs kept at room temp

- 1 1/4 teaspoon of Sweetleaf stevia drops

- 1 tablespoon of psyllium husks

- 1/4 teaspoon of salt preferably sea salt

Instructions

- Place the coconut oil and the unsweetened baking chocolate in some microwaveable bowl. Just microwave these until completely melted.

- Add stevia, monk fruit, eggs, and vanilla extract to the melted chocolate mixture then combine with the electric mixer.

- Stir in the unsweetened psyllium husks, cocoa, and salt.

- Spread into a parchment paper lined on an 8x8 baking pan.

- Bake these at 350°F for about 25 minutes then cool completely before you can slice.

Nutrients per one serving: Calories 140, Total Fats 15.3g, Cholesterol 15.3mg, Total Carbs 5g, Protein 3.3g

Fat bombs with sausage, ricotta, and parmesan

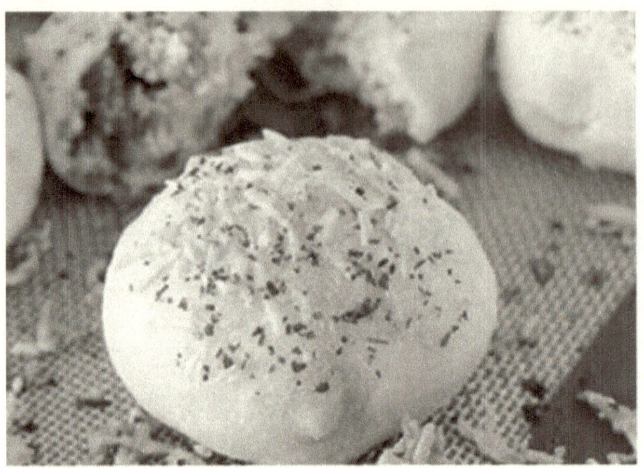

Servings 20

Total Time: 45 minutes

Ingredients:

*   200 g pizza dough

*   500 g pork sausage

*   ¼ tsp salt

*   ¼ tsp ground black pepper

*   ½ tsp dried parsley

*   ½ tsp dried basil

*   ½ tsp. of garlic powder

*   ¼ tsp sweet peppers

*   ¼ tsp oregano

*   ¼ tsp dried thyme

- 1 cup of young spinach

- 50 g ricotta cheese

- 100 g parmesan

- 1 egg

Cooking process:

1. Divide pizza dough into equal 10-12 parts.

2. Cut sausage into small cubes. Grate the cheese. Lay out sausage, herbs, and spices in a heated frying pan. Fry until golden color for 5 minutes.

3. Add spinach, ricotta and ¼ cup of Parmesan. Mix, and simmer for 5 minutes. To cool mix.

4. Preheat the oven to 200 °C. Roll out each dough part into a thin circle. To put 1 tablespoon of sausage stuffing in the center. To curtail edges so that to create round bomb.

5. Cover the baking sheet with parchment. Lay out ready bombs. Grease dough with beaten-up egg and sprinkle parmesan. Bake in an oven for 18 minutes.

Nutrients per one serving:

Calories: 340 | Fats: 24 g. | Carbohydrates: 4.5 g. | Proteins: 18 g.

Nutbutter Cup

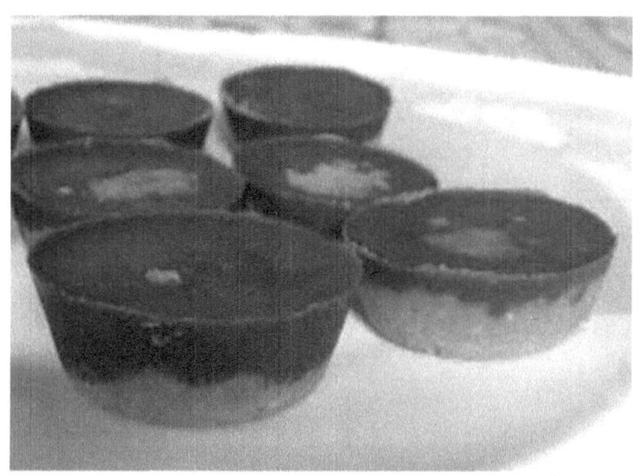

Serving: 12 people

Prep Time: 5 min

Cook Time: 5 min

Ingredients

- 2 packets of stevia, or 2 tablespoons of honey

- ½ teaspoon of unrefined sea salt

- ½ cup of thick nut butter

- ½ cup of softened butter or coconut oil

Instructions

- If the nut butter has been separated, ensure you mix oil in well or fat bombs will become too soft.

- Combine the nut butter, the softened butter or the coconut oil, stevia or the honey, and the sea salt in some small bowl using a fork, or in a food processor with a circular blade.

- If you are using silicone candy mold, place the mold on some tray or a large plate to transfer it to freezer easily after filling.

- Once it has been combined, pour this into silicone candy mold or parchment-lined loaf pan or a small casserole dish.

- Freeze for about 1 hour or until it becomes firm but not solid, then cut in 12 pieces.

- Store in a freezer covered then enjoy as desired!

Nutrients per one serving: Calories: 127, Saturated fat: 5, Fat: 13, Trans fat: 0, Sugar: 1, Sodium: 160 mg, Carbohydrates: 2, Fiber: 1, Cholesterol: 20 mg, Protein: 2

Spinach keto bombs

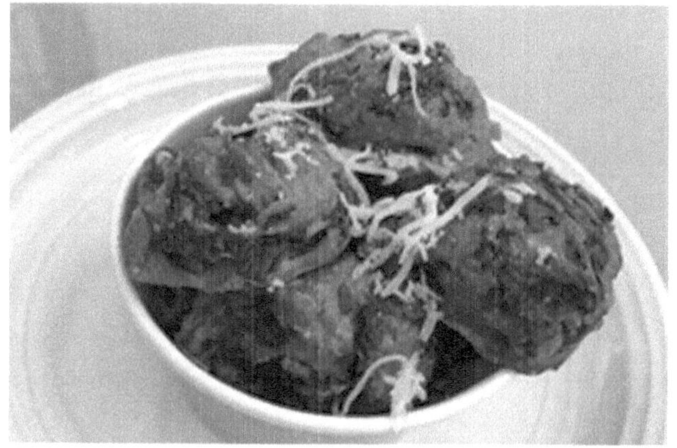

Servings 10

Total Time: 45 minutes

Ingredients:

- 5 cups fresh spinach leaves

- 50 g parmesan

- 3 eggs

- 1 tsp garlic powder

- 1 tsp Italian spices

- ½ tsp salt

- 3 tbsp breadcrumbs

Cooking process:

1. Preheat the oven to 180 °C.

2. In the saucepan boil the water and dip the leaves of spinach for 2 minutes. Recline into a colander and get rid of excess fluid.

3. In a bowl, mix spinach, grated Parmesan, eggs, garlic powder, spices,

salt, and breadcrumbs.

4.   Cover the baking sheet with parchment. Form balls with a tablespoon and lay out them on a baking sheet. Bake in the oven for 20 minutes. Increase the temperature to 200 degrees and leave them for next 10 minutes.

Nutrients per one serving:

Calories: 150 | Fats: 11 g. | Carbohydrates: 0.9 g. | Proteins: 16 g.

Cream Cheese Crab Dip

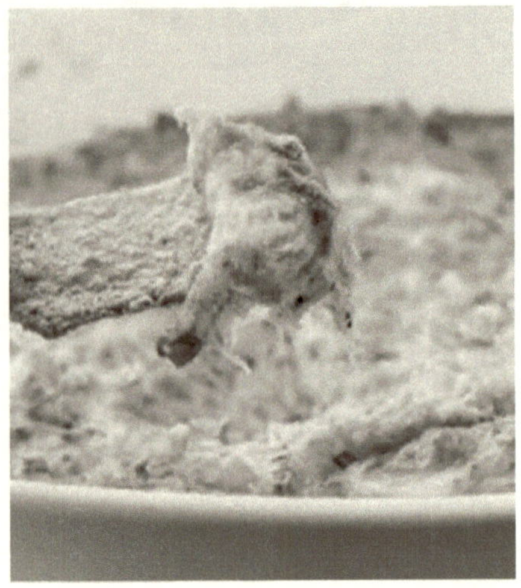

Serving: 12 people

Prep Time 5 min

Cook Time 30 min

Ingredients

- 1/2 teaspoon of garlic powder

- 1/2 teaspoon of onion powder

- 1/2 teaspoon of salt

- 1/4 teaspoon of dry mustard

- 8 ounces of lump crab meat

- 8 ounces of cream cheese softened

- 1/2 cup of avocado mayonnaise

- 1 tablespoon of lemon juice

- 1 teaspoon of Worcestershire sauce

- 1/4 teaspoon of black pepper

Instructions

- Combine all the ingredients into some small baking dish then spread out evenly.

- Bake them at 375°F for about 25-30 minutes.

- Enjoy with low carb crackers or some vegetables.

Nutrients per one serving: Calories 142, Total Fat 14.8g, Cholesterol 35mg, Protein 4.2g

Keto mozzarella sticks

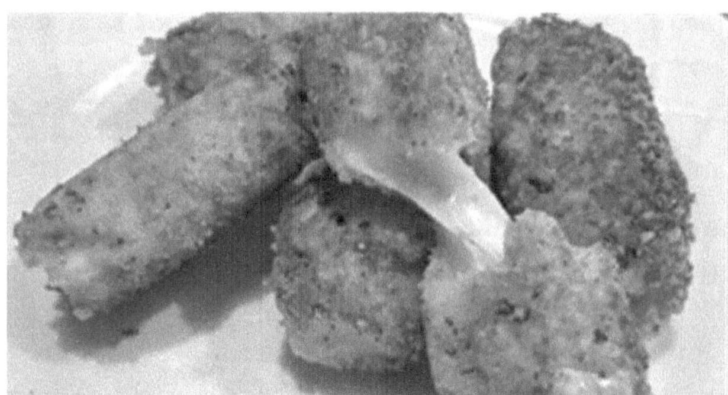

Servings 10

Total Time: 20 minutes + 20 minutes for freezing

Ingredients:

- 200 g mozzarella sticks

- 100 g parmesan

- 1 tbsp coconut flour

- 1 tsp baking powder

- ½ tsp garlic powder

- ½ tsp dried basil

- ½ tsp oregano

- 1 egg

- 2 tbsp olive oil

- A pinch of salt and ground black pepper

Cooking process:

1.   In a bowl, mix the egg, salt, and black pepper. In another container, mix coconut flour, garlic powder, dried herbs and grated parmesan.

2.   Roll each mozzarella stick in beaten egg and dry mix. Repeat twice to form a double breading.

3.   Lay out mozzarella on the dish and leave in the freezer for 20 minutes.

4.   Preheat the oil in a frying pan and fry the mozzarella sticks for 1 minute from all sides. Lay out on paper towels to remove excess oil. Serve with low-carb sauce.

Nutrients per one serving:

Calories: 390 | Fats: 28 g. | Carbohydrates: 3 g. | Proteins: 35 g.

Chapter 6: SWEET & SNACK FAT BOMBS RECIPES

LIQUID FAT BOMBS RECIPES

Blueberry Chocolate Smoothie

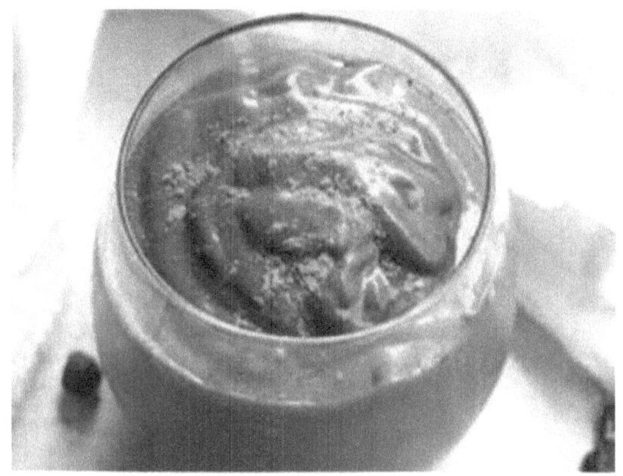

Serving: 1 serving

Prep Time: 5 min

Ingredients

- 1/2 (13.5-ounce) can of coconut milk

- 1 tablespoon of powdered unflavored gelatin

- 6 drops of liquid stevia

- 6 ice cubes

- 1 tablespoon of coconut oil, softened

- 1 tablespoon of cocoa powder

- 1/4 cup of frozen blueberries

Instructions

- Pour milk and the gelatin into your blender then blend so as to combine.

•   Add the remaining ingredients other than ice cubes then blend for another minute until it is well mixed.

•   Place the ice cubes into a blender then process until the smoothie thickens.

•   Serve immediately.

Nutrients per one serving: Calories: 560, Fat: 55g, Protein: 12g, Sodium: 41mg, Fiber: 5g, Carbohydrates: 16g, Sugar: 3g

Cinnamon Roll Smoothie

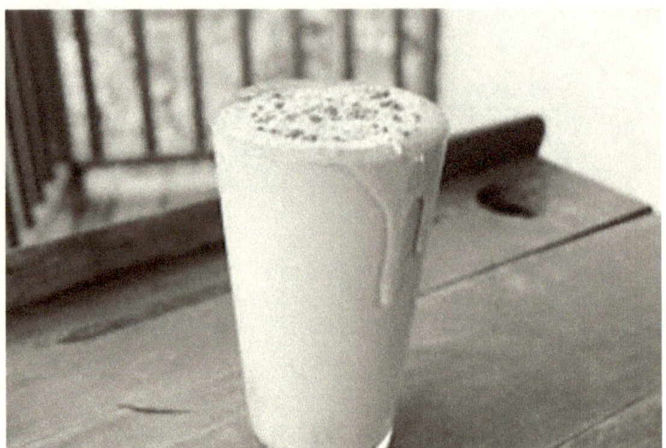

Serving: 1 fat bomb

Prep Time: 5 min

Ingredients

•   1/2 teaspoon and 1/8 teaspoon of cinnamon, divided

•   6 drops of liquid stevia

•   6 ice cubes

•   6 ounces of half-and-half

•   1 tablespoon of softened cream cheese

- 1 teaspoon of vanilla extract

Instructions

- Pour half-and-half and the cream cheese into some blender then blend to combine.

- Add 1/2 teaspoon cinnamon, vanilla and stevia then blend for another minute until they are well mixed.

- Place the ice cubes into a blender then process until the smoothie thickens.

- Sprinkle 1/8 teaspoon of cinnamon on the top and serve.

Nutrients per one serving: Calories: 283, Fat: 24g, Protein: 6g, Sodium: 116mg, Fiber: 1g, Carbohydrates: 9g, Sugar: 1g

Thai Iced Tea

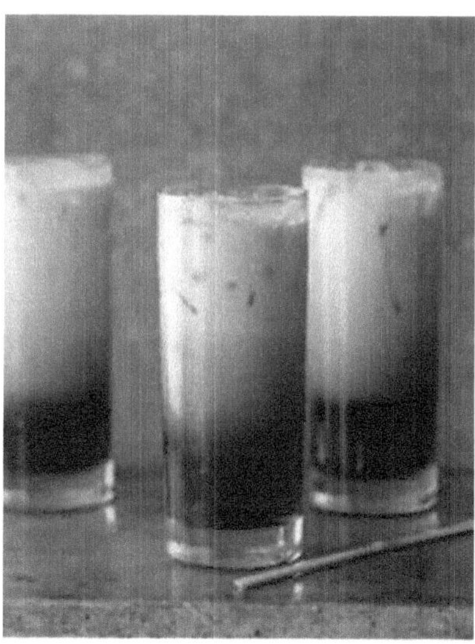

Serving: 2 fat bombs

Prep Time: 15 min

Cook Time: 8 min

Ingredients

- 4 cups of water

- 1 tablespoon of heavy cream

- 2 tablespoons of coconut milk

- 2 tablespoons of black tea leaves, Ceylon variety

- 2 crushed cardamom pods

- 1 teaspoon of star anise seeds

- 1 teaspoon of erythritol or granular of Swerve, or 2 drops of stevia glycerite

- 1/8 teaspoon of vanilla extract

Instructions

- In some small saucepan placed over high heat, bring some water to boil, and lower the heat to low.

- Add cardamom, tea leaves and the anise seeds then simmer for 3 minutes. Strain.

- Let the brewed tea to cool, and pour over the ice in some 2 tall glasses.

- In some small bowl combine cream, coconut milk, sweetener, and the vanilla then stir well until the sweetener has dissolved.

- Pour the cream mix on the top of the tea without stirring for the layers to remain separate.

- Serve immediately with tall spoon and straw.

Nutrients per one serving: Calories: 144, Fat: 15g, Protein: 1g, Sodium: 28mg, Fiber: 1g, Carbohydrates: 7g, Sugar: 0g

Caffeine-Free Coconut Vanilla Tea

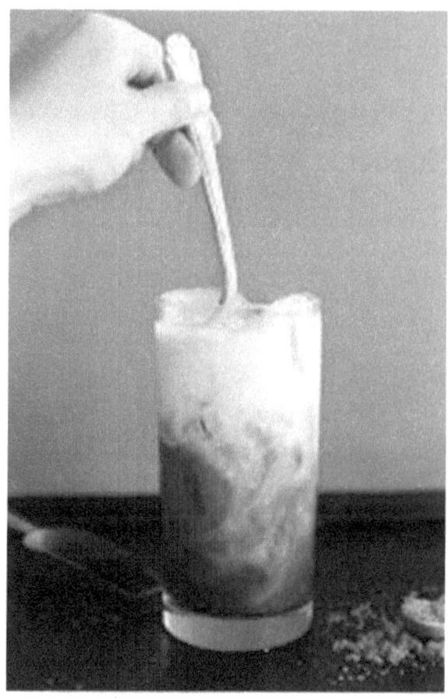

Serving: 1 serving

Prep Time: 2 min

Cook Time: 8 min

Ingredients

- 11/2 cups of hot water

- 1 tablespoon of coconut oil

- 1 teabag of rooibos tea

- 1 teaspoon of erythritol or granular of Swerve, or 2 drops of stevia glycerite

- 1/8 teaspoon of vanilla extract (optional)

Instructions

- Place a teabag in water then brew for about 8 minutes.

- Place the brewed tea in your blender with the remaining ingredients.

- Blend on high for 15 seconds.

- Serve immediately.

Nutrients per one serving: Calories: 135, Fat: 14g, Protein: 0g, Sodium: 11mg, Fiber: 0g, Carbohydrates: 8g, Sugar: 0g

Po Cha

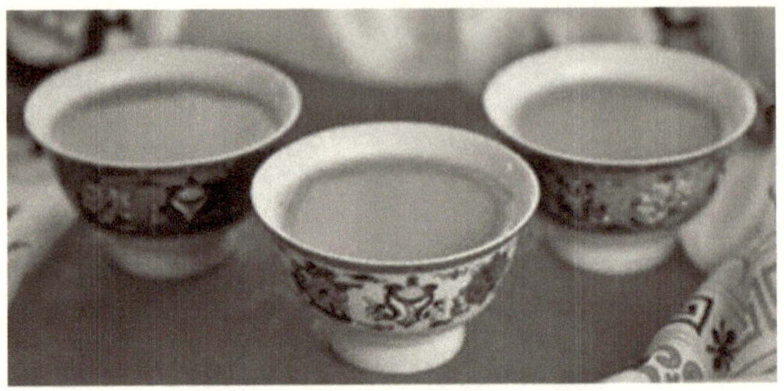

Serving: 2 people

Prep Time: 3 min

Cook Time: 8 min

Ingredients

- 2 tablespoons of heavy cream

- 1/8 teaspoon of sea salt

- 1 drop of smoke flavor

- 4 cups of water

- 2 tablespoons of black tea leaves

- 2 tablespoons of butter

Instructions

- In some small saucepan placed over high heat, just bring some water to a boil, and lower the heat to low.

- Add some tea leaves to the water then simmer for about 3 minutes and strain.

- Combine the brewed tea with the remaining ingredients in a blender then mix on high for about 3 minutes.

- Serve immediately.

Nutrients per one serving: Calories: 153, Fat: 17g, Protein: 0g, Sodium: 169mg, Fiber: 0g, Carbohydrates: 0g, Sugar: 0g

Creamy Coconut Smoothie

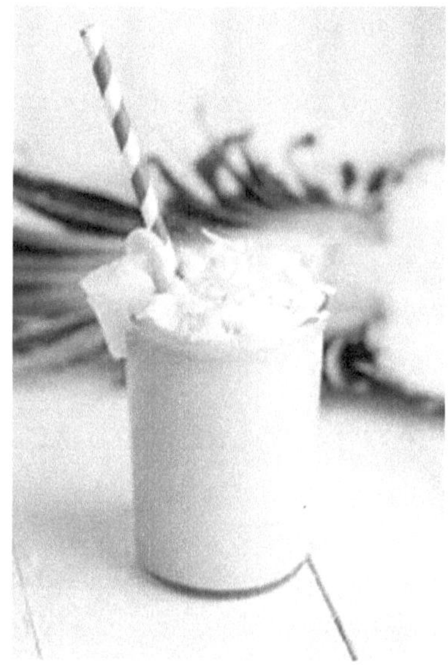

Serving: 1 fat bomb

Prep Time: 5 min

Ingredients

- 1/2 (13.5-ounce) can of coconut milk

- 1 tablespoon of unsweetened shredded coconut

- 6 drops of liquid stevia

- 1 tablespoon of powdered unflavored gelatin

- 1 tablespoon of softened coconut oil

- 1 teaspoon of vanilla extract

- 6 ice cubes

Instructions

- Pour milk and the gelatin into the blender then blend so as to combine.

- Add the remaining ingredients except for the ice cubes and blend for another minute until they are well mixed.

- Place the ice cubes into the blender then process until the smoothie thickens.

- Serve immediately.

Nutrients per one serving: Calories: 559, Fat: 57g, Protein: 10g, Sodium: 41mg, Fiber: 0g, Carbohydrates: 7g, Sugar: 1g

Creamy Mexican Hot Chocolate

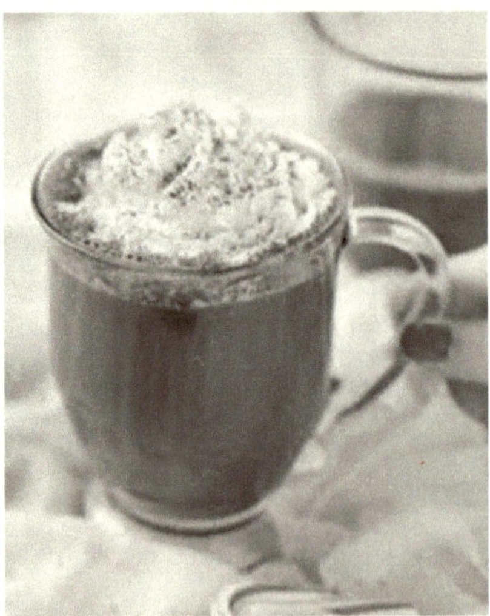

Serving: 2 people

Prep Time: 3 min

Cook Time: 5 min

Ingredients

*   1/8 teaspoon of vanilla extract

*   1 cup of water

*   1 cup of heavy cream

*   2 teaspoons of erythritol or granular of Swerve, or 2 drops of stevia glycerite

*   4 tablespoons of unsweetened whipped cream

*   1/3 cup of cocoa powder

*   1 teaspoon of cinnamon

Instructions

*   In some small saucepan placed over very low heat, just combine all the ingredients except the whipped cream.

*   Heat while stirring frequently until the cocoa powder is dissolved completely, for about 5 minutes. Avoid boiling.

*   When it's ready to serve, just pour the chocolate into 2 cups then top with the whipped cream.

Nutrients per one serving: Calories: 538, Fat: 56g, Protein: 6g, Sodium: 63mg, Fiber: 5g, Carbohydrates: 17g, Sugar: 0g

Eggnog Smoothie

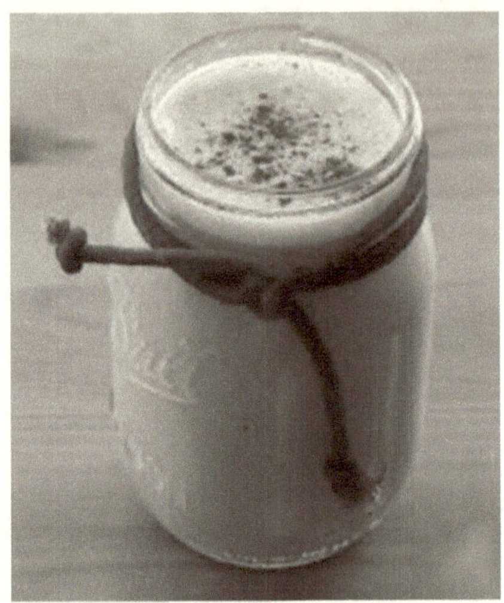

Serving: 2 fat bombs

Prep Time: 10 min

Ingredients

- 2 large eggs, the yolk and the white separated

- 8 ounces of heavy cream

- 8 drops of liquid stevia

- 1 tablespoon of granular Swerve

- 8 ice cubes

- 1⁄2 teaspoon of vanilla extract

- 1 teaspoon of nutmeg

- 1⁄8 teaspoon of ground cloves

- 3⁄8 teaspoon of cinnamon, divided

Instructions

•	In some medium bowl, beat the egg whites using a hand mixer until some stiff peaks form. Keep aside.

•	In some separate large bowl, beat the yolks using a mixer until the color changes to a pale yellow. Add vanilla, nutmeg, cream, cloves, 1/8 teaspoon cinnamon, the stevia, and the Swerve then stir well to combine.

•	Fold the whites into the yolk mixture.

•	Pour mix into the blender with the ice cubes then blend until the mixture thickens.

•	Sprinkle 1/8 teaspoon of cinnamon on the top of every glass then serve immediately.

Nutrients per one serving: Calories: 468, Fat: 47g, Protein: 9g, Sodium: 113mg, Fiber: 1g, Carbohydrates: 5g, Sugar: 1g

Gingerbread Gem Smoothie

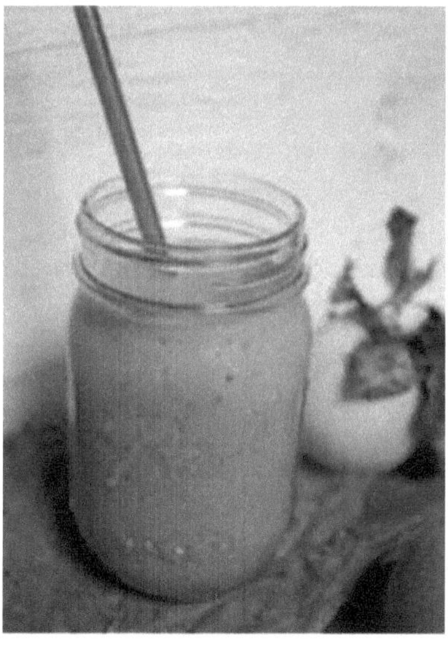

Serving: 1 fat bomb

Prep Time: 5 min

Ingredients

- 1⁄2 teaspoon of ground ginger

- 1⁄2 teaspoon of cinnamon

- 6 drops of liquid stevia

- 6 ice cubes

- 6 ounces of unsweetened almond milk

- 1 tablespoon of powdered unflavored gelatin

- 1 tablespoon of almond butter

- 1⁄2 teaspoon of vanilla extract

Instructions

- Pour the milk and the gelatin into your blender then blend to combine.

- Add the remaining ingredients except the ice cubes then blend for an extra minute until they are well mixed.

- Place the ice cubes into a blender then process until the smoothie thickens.

- Serve immediately.

Nutrients per one serving: Calories: 221, Fat: 11g, Protein: 16g, Sodium: 174mg, Fiber: 3g, Carbohydrates: 16g, Sugar: 9g

Key Lime Pie Smoothie

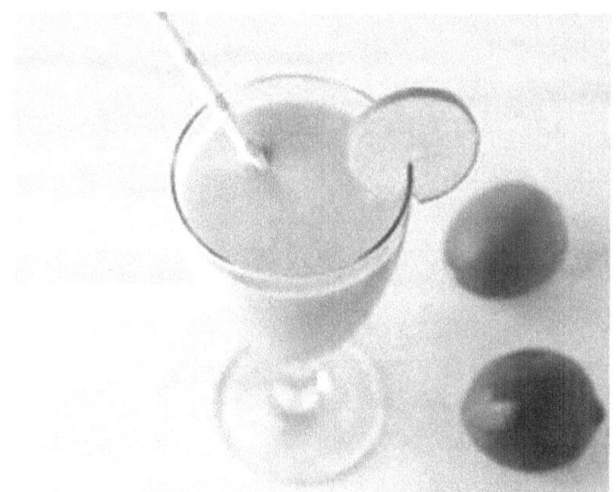

Serving: 1 fat bomb

Prep Time: 5 min

Ingredients

- 1 teaspoon of lime zest

- 6 drops of liquid stevia

- 6 ice cubes

- 6 ounces of half-and-half

- 1 tablespoon of powdered unflavored gelatin

- 1 teaspoon of vanilla extract

- 2 tablespoons of freshly squeezed key lime juice

Instructions

- Pour the half-and-half and the gelatin into some blender then blend so as to combine.

- Add the remaining ingredients other than the ice cubes then blend for an extra minute until they are well mixed.

- Place the ice cubes into the blender then process until the smoothie thickens.

- Serve immediately.

Nutrients per one serving: Calories: 280, Fat: 20g, Protein: 12g, Sodium: 91mg, Fiber: 2g, Carbohydrates: 17g, Sugar: 3g

Matcha Madness Smoothie

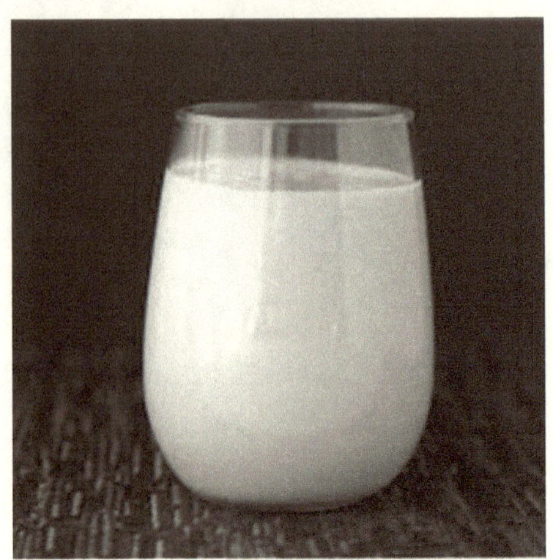

Serving: 1 fat bomb

Prep Time: 5 min

Ingredients

- 1/2 (13.5-ounce) can of coconut milk

- 1 tablespoon of matcha

- 6 drops of liquid stevia

- Ice cubes

- 1 tablespoon of powdered unflavored gelatin

- 2 tablespoons of almond butter

- 1 teaspoon of vanilla extract

Instructions

- Pour milk and the gelatin into your blender then blend to combine.

- Add the remaining ingredients other than the ice cubes then blend for an extra minute until it is well mixed.

- Place the ice cubes into a blender then process until the smoothie thickens.

- Serve immediately.

Nutrients per one serving: Calories: 610, Fat: 57g, Protein: 19g, Sodium: 187mg, Fiber: 4g, Carbohydrates: 15g, Sugar: 4g

Peanut Butter Cup Smoothie

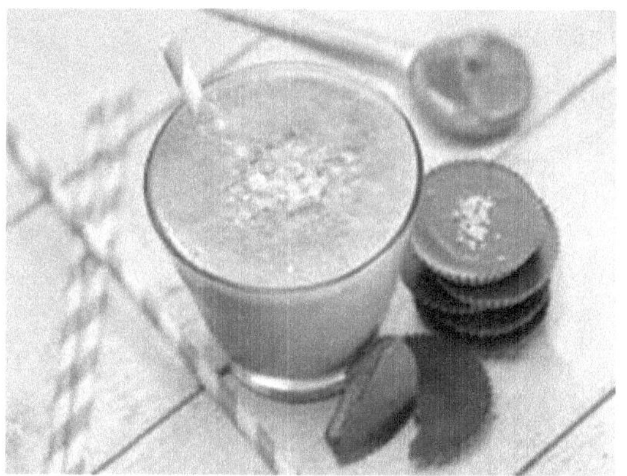

Serving: 1 fat bomb

Prep Time: 5 min

Ingredients

- 2 tablespoons of cocoa powder

- 1 teaspoon of vanilla extract

- 6 drops of liquid stevia

- Ice cubes

*   1/2 (13.5-ounce) can of coconut milk

*   1 tablespoon of powdered unflavored gelatin

*   2 tablespoons of peanut butter

Instructions

*   Pour the milk and the gelatin into your blender then blend well to combine.

*   Add the remaining ingredients other than the ice cubes then blend for an extra minute until they are well mixed.

*   Place the ice cubes into the blender then process until the smoothie thickens.

*   Serve immediately.

Nutrients per one serving: Calories: 622, Fat: 58g, Protein: 20g, Sodium: 189mg, Fiber: 6g, Carbohydrates: 18g, Sugar: 4g

Thai Iced Coffee

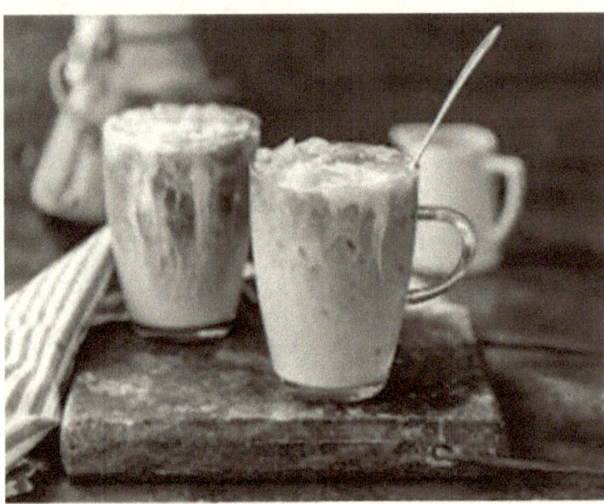

Ingredients

*   4 cups of cooled strong brewed coffee

*   1/8 teaspoon of vanilla extract

- 4 tablespoons of heavy cream

- 4 teaspoons of erythritol or granular of Swerve, or 3 drops of stevia glycerite

- 2 tablespoons of coconut milk

Instructions

- Pour the coffee into some large bowl then mix with coconut milk, sweetener, and vanilla.

- Pour the coffee mixture over the ice in some 2 tall glasses.

- Pour the cream on the top of the coffee without stirring for the layers to remain separate.

- Serve immediately using some tall spoon and straw.

Nutrients per one serving: Calories: 548, Fat: 15g, Protein: 22g, Sodium: 77mg, Fiber: 0g, Carbohydrates: 80g, Sugar: 0g

Tibetan Butter Tea

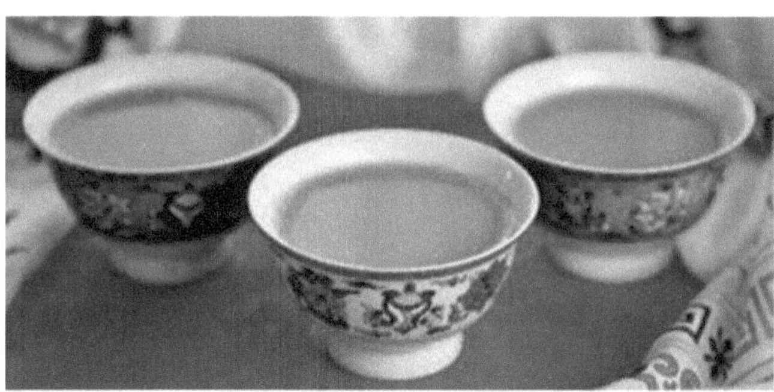

Serving: 2 fat bombs

Prep Time: 3 min

Cook Time: 8 min

Ingredients

- 4 cups of water

- 1/8 teaspoon of sea salt

- Drop smoke of flavor

- 2 tablespoons of black tea leaves

- 2 tablespoons of butter

- 2 tablespoons of heavy cream

Instructions

- In some small saucepan placed over high heat, bring the water to boil, then lower the heat to low.

- Add the tea leaves to the water then simmer for 3 minutes. Strain.

- Combine the brewed tea with the remaining ingredients in some blender then mix on high for about 3 minutes.

- Serve immediately.

Nutrients per one serving: Calories: 153, Fat: 17g, Protein: 0g, Sodium: 169mg, Fiber: 0g, Carbohydrates: 0g, Sugar: 0g

Coconut Coffee

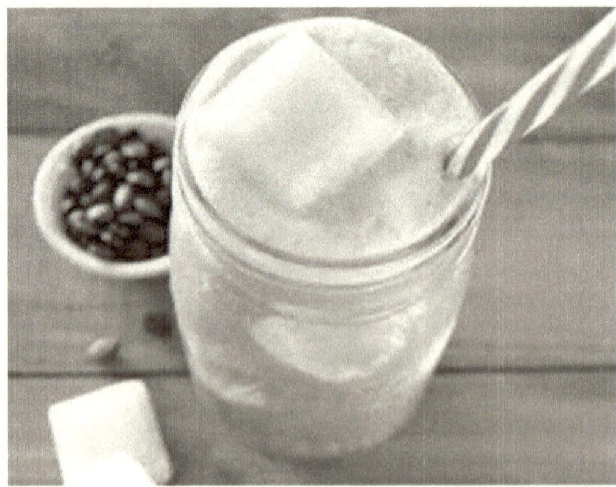

Serving: 1 fat bomb

Prep Time: 1 min

Ingredients

*   11/2 cups of hot brewed coffee

*   2 teaspoons of erythritol or granular of Swerve, or 2 drops of stevia glycerite

*   1 tablespoon of coconut oil

*   1 tablespoon of butter

*   1/8 teaspoon of sea salt

Instructions

*   Place all the ingredients in some blender.

*   Blend on high for about 15 seconds.

*   Serve immediately.

Nutrients per one serving: Calories: 534, Fat: 28g, Protein: 16g, Sodium: 344mg, Fiber: 0g, Carbohydrates: 61g, Sugar: 0g

Orange Delight Smoothie

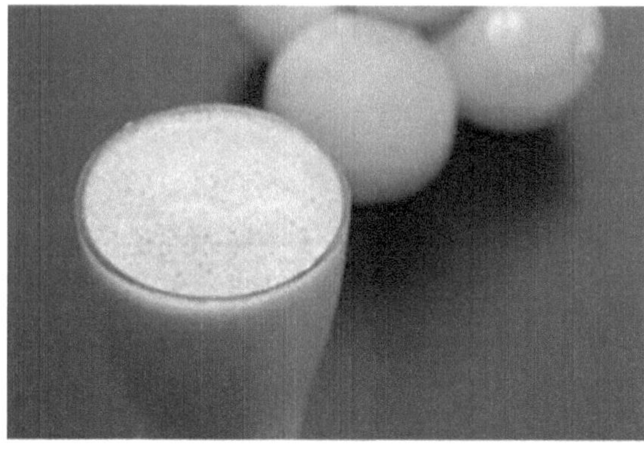

Ingredients

*   6 ounces of half-and-half

*   Drops of liquid stevia

*   6 ice cubes

*   Tablespoon of powdered unflavored gelatin

*   1 teaspoon of vanilla extract

*   2 tablespoons of orange juice, freshly squeezed

*   1 teaspoon of orange zest

Instructions

*   Pour the half-and-half and the gelatin into your blender then blend to combine.

*   Add the remaining ingredients other than the ice cubes then blend for an extra minute until they are well mixed.

*   Place the ice cubes into the blender then process until the smoothie thickens.

*   Serve immediately.

Nutrients per one serving: Calories: 271, Fat: 19g, Protein: 11g, Sodium: 84mg, Fiber: 0g, Carbohydrates: 12g, Sugar: 4g

Amaretto Chilled Coffee

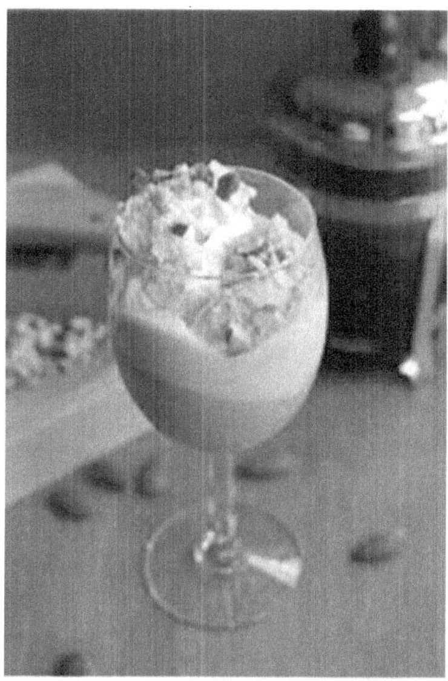

Serving: 2 fat bombs

Prep Time: 8 min

Ingredients

*   2 cups of cooled brewed coffee

*   1/2 cup of chilled heavy cream

*   1 teaspoon crumbled roasted almonds

*   4 teaspoons of erythritol or granular Swerve /3 drops of stevia glycerite, divided

*   4 drops of divided amaretto flavor

Instructions

*   Pour coffee into some medium bowl then mix with half of sweetener and half of amaretto flavor.

*   In your blender add the chilled cream, the remaining amaretto flavor, and the remaining sweetener, then blend on high till the cream is whipped.

• Once it is ready to serve, just pour the coffee mixture over the ice in 2 glasses.

• Spoon the whipped cream on the top of the coffee mix. Decorate using chopped almonds.

• Serve immediately using a spoon and straw.

Nutrients per one serving: Calories: 421, Fat: 23g, Protein: 12g, Sodium: 55mg, Fiber: 0g, Carbohydrates: 45g, Sugar: 0g

Vanilla Smoothie

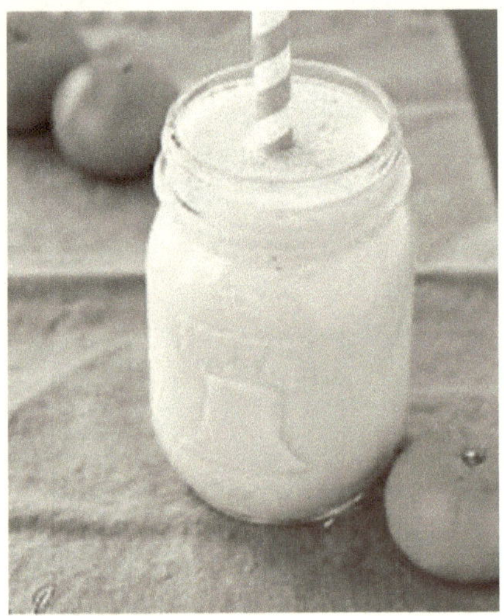

Serving: 1 fat bomb

Prep Time: 5 min

Ingredients

• The pulp of 1 vanilla bean, scraped

• 4 drops of liquid stevia

• 6 ice cubes

• 6 ounces of half-and-half

- 1 tablespoon of powdered unflavored gelatin

- 1 teaspoon of vanilla extract

Instructions

- Pour the half-and-half and the gelatin into your blender then blend to combine.

- Add the remaining ingredients other than the ice cubes then blend for an extra minute until they are well mixed.

- Place the ice cubes into the blender then process until the smoothie thickens.

- Serve immediately.

Nutrients per one serving: Calories: 274, Fat: 19g, Protein: 11g, Sodium: 83mg, Fiber: 0g, Carbohydrates: 8g, Sugar: 1g

Liquid Fat Bomb Smoothie

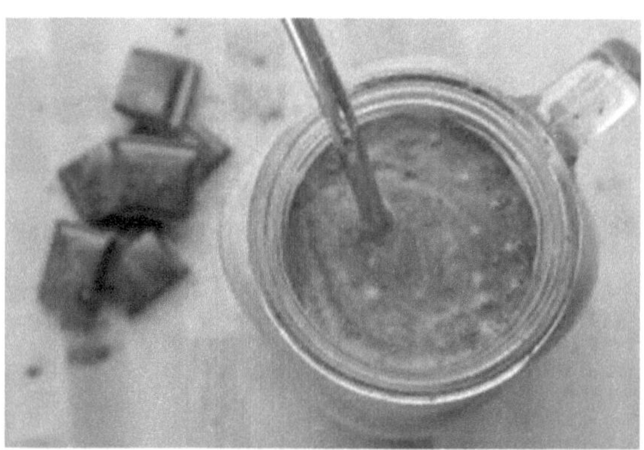

Ingredients

- 1 cup of full-fat coconut milk

- 2/3 cup of frozen berries

- 1/4 cup of water

- 2 raw egg yolks

*   1 scoop of whey protein

Instructions

*   Add all the ingredients into your blender then blend well until smooth. Enjoy!

Nutrients per one serving: Total Fat: 70 grams, Saturated Fat: 50 grams, Carbohydrate: 27 grams, Protein: 27 grams, Total Calories: 840

Keto Fat Bomb Smoothie

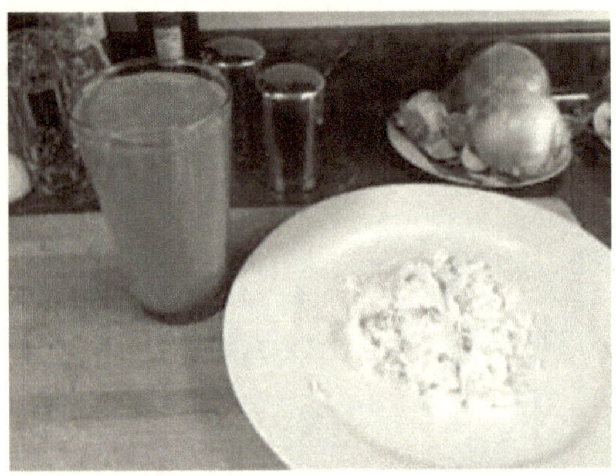

Ingredients

*   1 Cup of Coconut Milk

*   1/2 tsp of Cinnamon

*   1/2 Cup of Ice

*   2 tbsps. of Coconut Oil

*   1 tbsp. of Peanut Butter

*   1/2 tsp of Vanilla Extract

Instructions

*   Beginning with the ice, just add all the ingredients into your blender.

*   Blend well until smooth, then drink. You refrigerate for a later use,

though you can have to remix ingredients using a spoon after settling.

Nutrients per one serving: Calories 883, Protein 9g, Fat 79g, Carbs 17g

Avocado Almond Smoothie

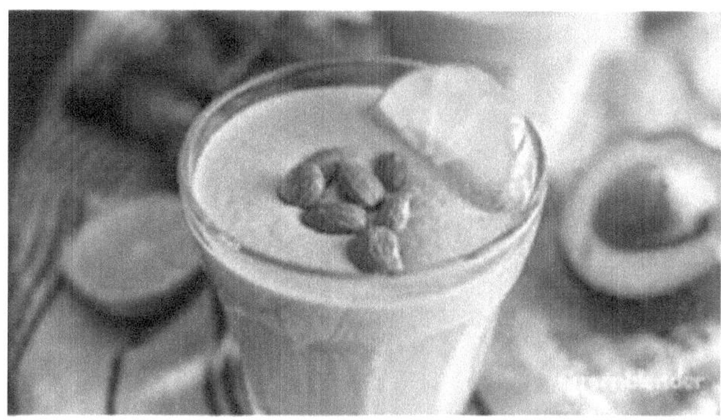

Serving: 2 fat bombs

Prep Time: 3 min

Ingredients

- 1 teaspoon of almond extract

- 4 drops of liquid stevia

- 2 tablespoons of coconut butter

- 1/2 pitted and peeled large avocado

- 1 cup of coconut milk

- 1/4 cup of ice

Instructions

- Combine all the ingredients in a blender then blend until they are smooth.

- Serve immediately.

Nutrients per one serving: Calories: 423, Fat: 45g, Protein: 3g, Sodium:

18mg, Fiber: 3g, Carbohydrates: 7g, Sugar: 0g

Vanilla Avocado Smoothie

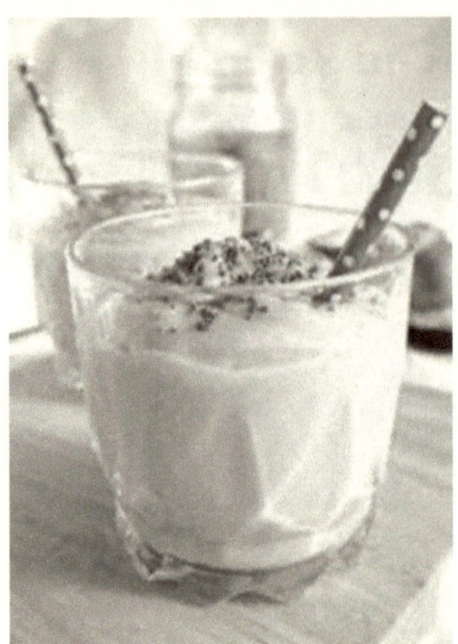

Serving: 1 fat bomb

Prep Time: 5 min

Ingredients

*   1⁄2 (13.5-ounce) can of coconut milk

*   1 teaspoon of vanilla extract

*   6 drops of liquid stevia

*   4 ice cubes

*   1 tablespoon of powdered unflavored gelatin

*   1 tablespoon of ground flaxseed

*   1⁄2 pitted and peeled medium avocado

Instructions

*   Pour gelatin, milk, and flaxseed into the blender then blend to

combine.

• Add the remaining ingredients other than the ice cubes then blend for an extra minute until they are well mixed.

• Place the ice cubes into the blender then process until the smoothie thickens.

• Serve immediately.

Nutrients per one serving: Calories: 603, Fat: 57g, Protein: 14g, Sodium: 46mg, Fiber: 9g, Carbohydrates: 17g, Sugar: 1g

Blueberry Chia Smoothie

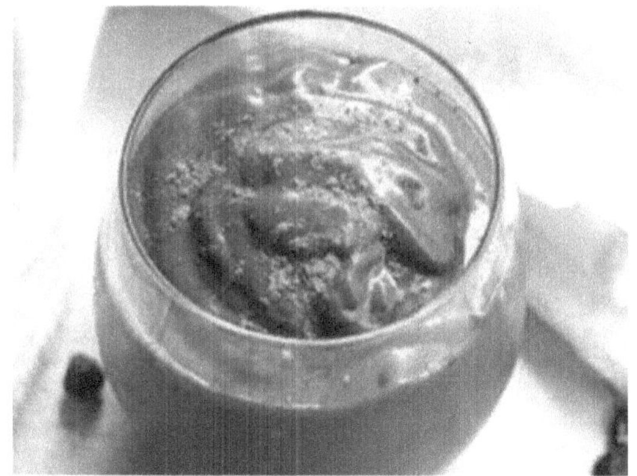

Ingredients

• 1 Cup of Hazelnut Milk

• Dash of Cinnamon or nutmeg

• 1 Cup of Frozen Blueberries

• 1 tbsp. of Cocoa Powder

• 1 Tsp of Chia Seeds

Instructions

• Place milk, berries, powder and the other ingredients in your blender and blend.

*   Add the milk first to ensure that powders don't get stuck to the bottom of your blender.

Nutrients per one serving: Calories 225, Protein 5g, Fat 6g, Carbs 45g

Vanilla Almond Butter Smoothie

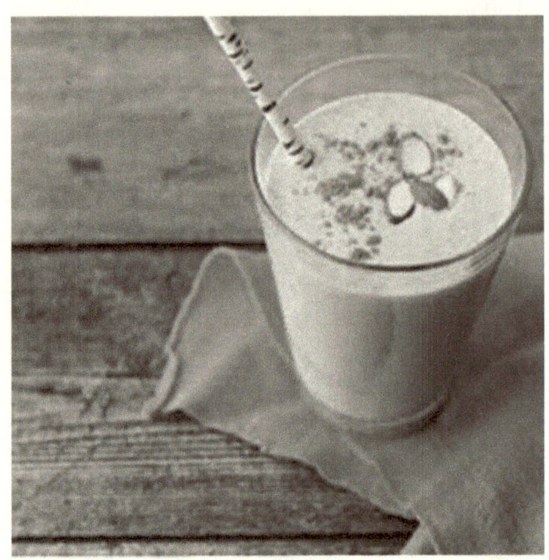

Serving: 1 fat bomb

Prep Time: 5 min

Ingredients

*   6 ounces of unsweetened almond milk

*   1/4 teaspoon of almond extract (optional)

*   6 drops of liquid stevia

*   Ice cubes

*   1 tablespoon of powdered unflavored gelatin

*   2 tablespoons of almond butter

*   1 teaspoon of vanilla extract

Instructions

- Pour the milk and the gelatin into some blender then blend so as to combine.

- Add the remaining ingredients other than the ice cubes then blend for an extra minute until they are well mixed.

- Place the ice cubes into the blender then process until the smoothie thickens.

- Serve immediately.

Nutrients per one serving: Calories: 316, Fat: 19g, Protein: 19g, Sodium: 248mg, Fiber: 3g, Carbohydrates: 17g, Sugar: 10g

Strawberry Vanilla Smoothie

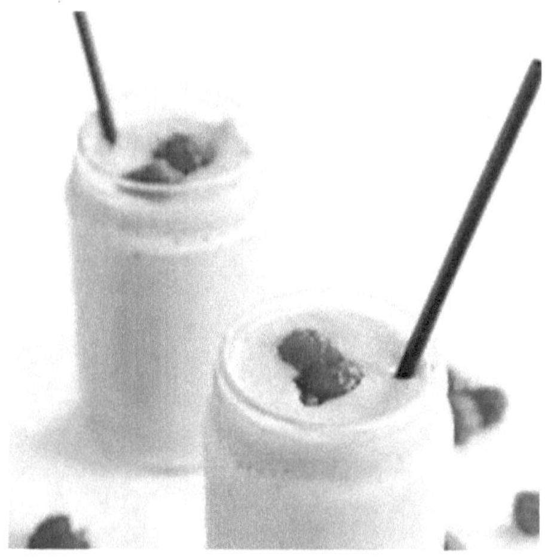

Serving: 1 fat bomb

Prep Time: 5 min

Ingredients

- 1/2 (13.5-ounce) can of coconut milk

- 1/4 cup of chopped fresh strawberries

- 6 drops of liquid stevia

- Tablespoon of powdered unflavored gelatin

- 1 tablespoon of softened coconut oil

- 1 teaspoon of vanilla extract

- 6 ice cubes

Instructions

- Pour the milk and the gelatin into the blender then blend to combine.

- Add the remaining ingredients other than the ice cubes then blend for an extra minute until they are well mixed.

- Place the ice cubes into the blender then process until the smoothie thickens.

- Serve immediately.

Nutrients per one serving: Calories: 540, Fat: 54g, Protein: 10g, Sodium: 39mg, Fiber: 1g, Carbohydrates: 9g, Sugar: 2g

Weight Cutting Berry Smoothie

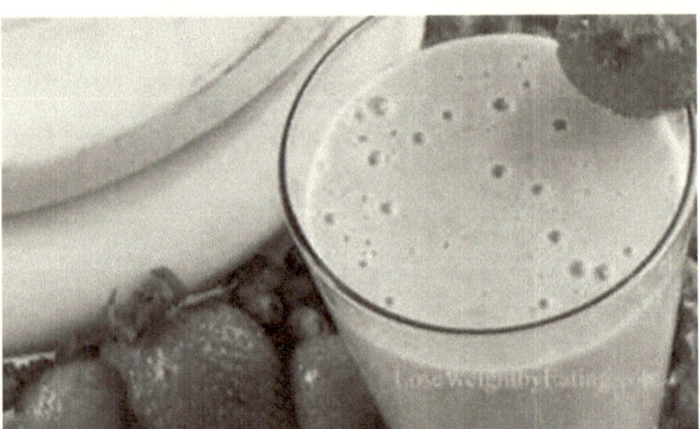

Ingredients

- 2 Cups Almond Milk

- 10 Strawberries

- 10 Raspberries

*   20 Blueberries

Instructions

*   Put in a blender, then blend and drink.

Nutrients per one serving: Calories 131, Vitamin C 154%, Vitamin D 50%, Vitamin E 44%, Calcium 92%

High Calorie Green Smoothie

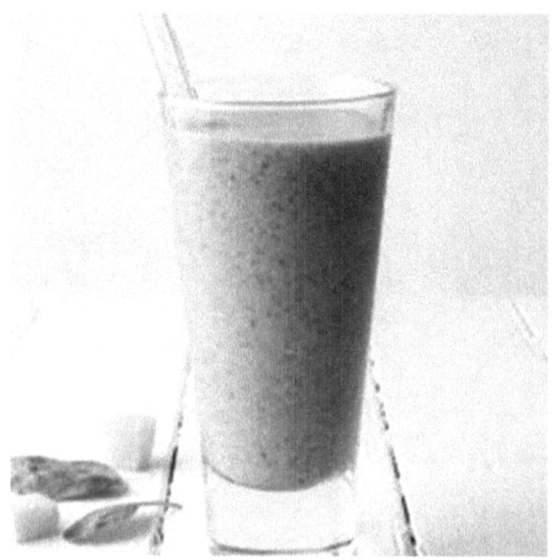

Ingredients

*   1/2 Cup of Spinach

*   1 Cup of Goat Milk

*   2 Bananas

*   1/2 Cup of Kale

*   1/2 Avocado

*   2 tbsps. of Macadamia Butter

*   2 tbsps. of Hemp Oil

Instructions

- Peel bananas

- Remove their skin then pit from avocado half.

- Place everything into your blender, then blend and enjoy.

Nutrients per one serving: Calories 1016, Protein 20, Fat 73, Carbs 81

Ultra Thick Bodybuilding Shake

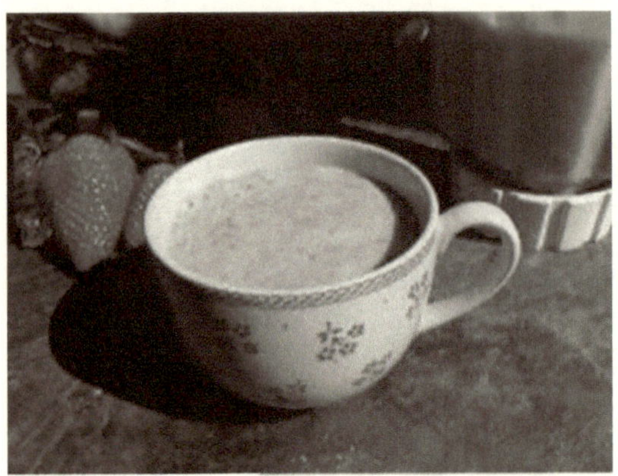

Ingredients

- 1/2 cup of oats

- 1 scoop of protein powder

- 1/2 cup of whole milk

- 1 frozen of banana

2 tbsps. of peanut butter

Instructions

- Blend oats into your powder.

- Add milk then mix oat powder with milk.

- After that add protein powder than the rest of the ingredients.

- Blend well until smooth.

- Drink.

Nutrients per one serving: Calories 142, Protein 66g, Carbs 102g, Fat 26g

Strawberry Coconut Smoothie

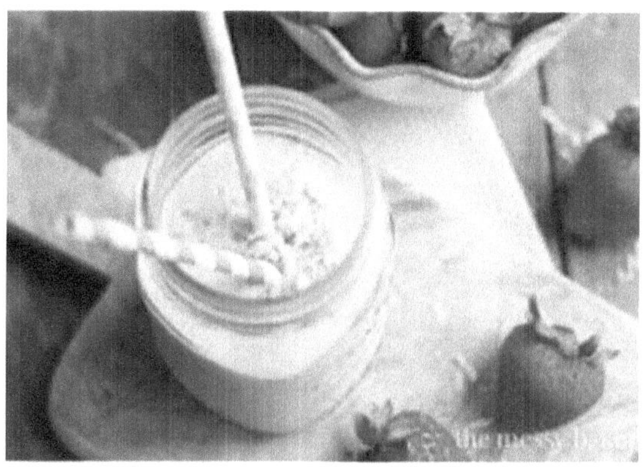

Ingredients

- 1 Cup of Coconut Milk

- 5 Strawberries

- 1/2 Cup of Ice

- 1/4 Cup of Heavy Cream

- 2 Tbsps. of Sugar-Free Vanilla syrup

Instructions

- Remove the stems from strawberries, then place all in your blender and blend.

Nutrients per one serving: Calories 299, Protein 2, Fat 27, Carbs 12

Basic High-Calorie Shake

Ingredients

- 1/2 Cup of Oats

- 1 Scoop of Protein

- 1 Banana

- 1/2 Cup of Milk

- 1/2 Cup of Half and Half

- 1 Tbsp. of Peanut Butter

Instructions

- Blend it, then drink it up.

Nutrients per one serving: Calories 702, Protein 39, Fat 29, Carbs 57.

Coffee Hazelnut Coconut

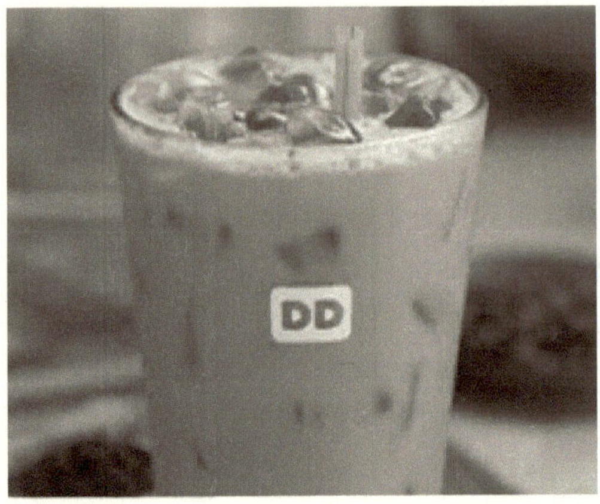

Serving: 12 fat bombs

Prep Time: 3 hours

Cook Time: 5 minutes

Ingredients

- 1/4 cup of coconut oil

* 1 tablespoon of cocoa powder

* 12 hazelnuts

* 1/4 cup of almond butter

* 1 tsp of instant coffee granules

* 12 drops of liquid stevia

Instructions

* Combine almond butter, coffee, coconut oil and the stevia in some small saucepan placed over medium heat, while stirring frequently until the ingredients melt. Turn off heat.

* Add the cocoa powder then stir well so as to combine.

* Pour the mixture into 12 molds for each to be about 2/3 full.

* Place a hazelnut into every filled mold.

* Freeze until set, then serve from the freezer.

Nutrients per one serving: Calories: 96, Fat: 8g, Protein: 2g, Sodium: 25mg, Fiber: 1g, Carbohydrates: 2g, Sugar: 1g

FROZEN FAT BOMBS RECIPES

Salted Caramel Almond

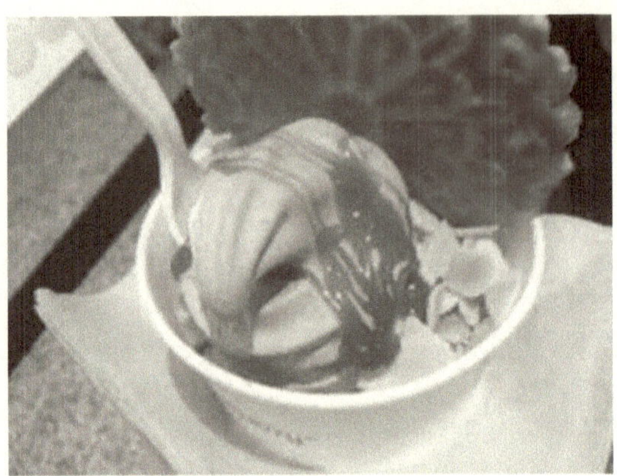

Serving: 12 fat bombs

Prep Time: 3 hours

Cook Time: 5 minutes

Ingredients

- 1/4 cup of granular Swerve

- 2 teaspoons of vanilla extract

- 12 whole almonds

- 1/4 cup of butter

- 1 teaspoon of coarse sea salt

Instructions

- Combine Swerve, butter, and vanilla in some small saucepan placed over medium heat, while stirring frequently until the ingredients melt. Turn off heat.

- Place 1 almond to each mold of 12-mold silicone candy tray.

- Pour the mixture over every almond until the molds become about 3/4 full.

- Sprinkle salt on the top of every fat bomb.

- Freeze until set, then serve from the freezer.

Nutrients per one serving: Calories: 64, Fat: 7g, Protein: 0g, Sodium: 296mg, Fiber: 0g, Carbohydrates: 1g, Sugar: 0g

Orange Creamsicle

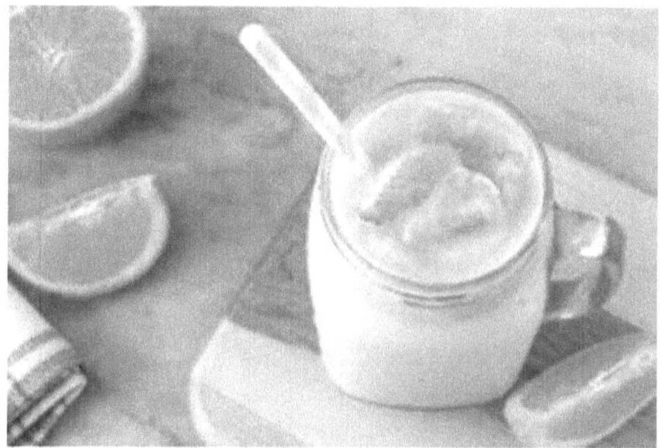

Serving: 12 fat bombs

Prep Time: 3 hours

Ingredients

- 1/4 cup of coconut oil

- 1/4 cup of heavy whipping cream

- 2 ounces of cream cheese, softened

- 2 tablespoons of orange juice

- 1 tablespoon of orange zest

- 12 drops of liquid stevia

Instructions

- Combine ingredients in some small wide-mouthed jar or in a bowl then blend with immersion blender, for about 30 seconds.

- Spread the mixture into your 12 molds of silicone candy mold tray.

- Freeze until set then serves from the freezer.

Nutrients per one serving: Calories: 75, Fat: 8g, Protein: 0g, Sodium: 17mg, Fiber: 0g, Carbohydrates: 1g, Sugar: 0g

Maca-Nutty Bites

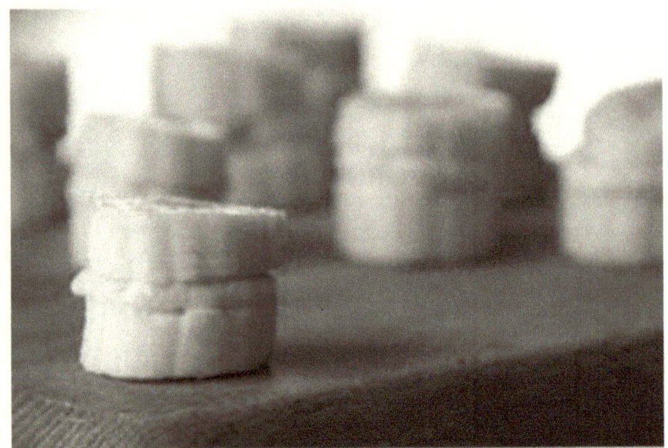

Serving: 12 fat bombs

Prep Time: 3 hours

Cook Time: 5 minutes

Ingredients

- 1/4 cup of coconut oil

- 1 tbsp. of cocoa powder

- 12 whole macadamia nuts

- 1/4 cup of almond butter

- 1 tsp of vanilla extract

- 12 drops of liquid stevia

Instructions

- Combine coconut oil, vanilla, almond butter and stevia in some small saucepan placed over medium heat, while stirring frequently till the ingredients melt. Turn off the heat.

- Add the cocoa powder then stir well so as to combine.

- Pour the mixture into 12 molds until each is about 2/3 full.

- Place a macadamia nut into every filled mold.

- Freeze until set, then serve from the freezer.

Nutrients per one serving: Calories: 93, Fat: 9g Protein: 2g, Sodium: 25mg, Fiber: 1g, Carbohydrates: 2g, Sugar: 1g

Almond Choco-Nut

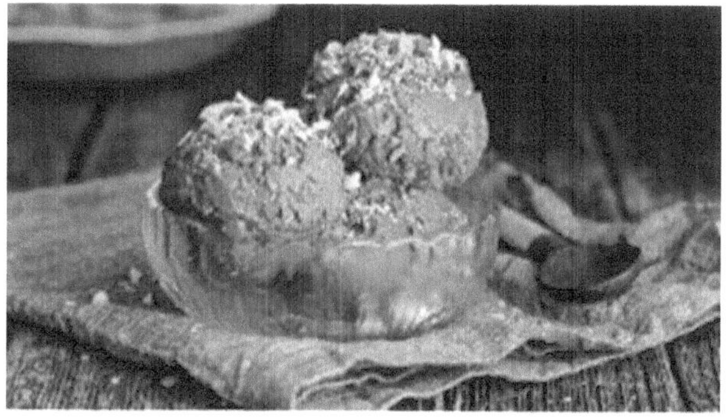

Serving: 12 fat bombs

Prep Time: 3 hours

Cook Time: 5 minutes

Ingredients

- 1/4 cup of coconut oil

- 1/4 cup of almonds

- 1 tablespoon of shredded coconut

- 1/4 cup of almond butter

- 12 drops of liquid stevia

- 2 tablespoons of cocoa powder

Instructions

- Combine almond butter, coconut oil and stevia in some small pot placed over medium heat, while stirring frequently until the ingredients have melted, then turn off heat.

- Add the cocoa powder and the almonds then stir well so as to combine.

- Pour the mixture into the 12 molds of ice cube tray or the silicone candy mold tray to be about 3/4 full.

- Sprinkle the shredded coconut on the top of every fat bomb.

- Freeze well until set. Serve from a freezer.

Nutrients per one serving: Calories: 87, Fat: 8g, Protein: 2g, Sodium: 25mg, Fiber: 1g, Carbohydrates: 2g, Sugar: 1g

Matcha Cream

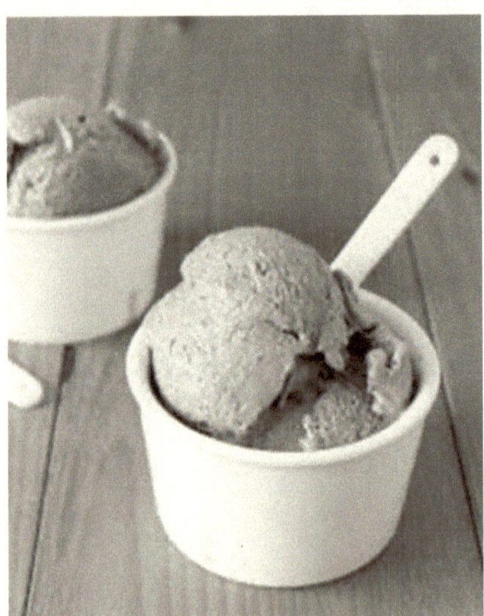

Serving: 12 fat bombs

Prep Time: 3–12 hours

Cook Time: 5 minutes

Ingredients

Ganache

*   1/2 teaspoon of matcha

*   2 tablespoons of confectioners Swerve

*   2 drops of stevia glycerite

*   3 ounces of cocoa butter

*   3 ounces of coconut cream

*   1 tablespoon of coconut oil

*   1/8 teaspoon of sea salt

Coating

*   2 tablespoons of matcha

Instructions

*   In some small double boiler placed over medium-low heat, just melt the cocoa butter as you stir slowly.

*   Add coconut cream, 1/2 teaspoon matcha, coconut oil, Swerve, the stevia, and the sea salt then mix well until they are incorporated.

*   Remove from the heat then continue stirring for about 10 seconds.

*   Pour into the silicone mold for the chocolate or the candy in the desired shape.

*   Freeze for about 3 hours. Once frozen, remove the shapes from the molds and sprinkle with about 2 tablespoons of matcha so as to coat tops.

- They may be stored in some sealed container in a freezer or a refrigerator.

Nutrients per one serving: Calories: 103, Fat: 9g, Protein: 0g, Sodium: 291mg, Fiber: 0g, Carbohydrates: 6g, Sugar: 5g

Coconut Rum

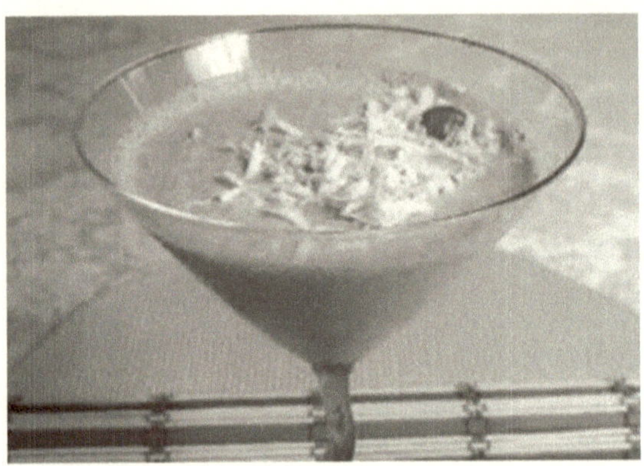

Serving: 10 fat bombs

Prep Time: 5 hours

Cook Time: 5 min

Ingredients

Ganache

- 2 ounces of cocoa butter

- 2 ounces of coconut cream

- 2 tablespoons of confectioners Swerve

- 1/4 teaspoon of rum flavor

- 2 drops of stevia glycerite

- 4 tablespoons of unsweetened shredded coconut

Coating

- 2 tablespoons of shredded coconut

Instructions

- In some small double boiler placed over medium-low heat, just melt the cocoa butter as you stir slowly.

- Add Swerve, rum flavor, coconut cream, stevia, and some 4 tablespoons of shredded coconut then mix well until well incorporated.

- Remove from the heat then keep on stirring for about 10 seconds.

- Pour into the silicone mold for the chocolate or the candy in the desired shape.

- Freeze for about 3 hours. Once frozen, just remove the ganache shapes from the molds then sprinkle using 2 tablespoons of shredded coconut so as to coat tops.

Nutrients per one serving: Calories: 86, Fat: 8g, Protein: 0g, Sodium: 3mg, Fiber: 0g, Carbohydrates: 5g, Sugar: 5g

Coconut White Chocolate

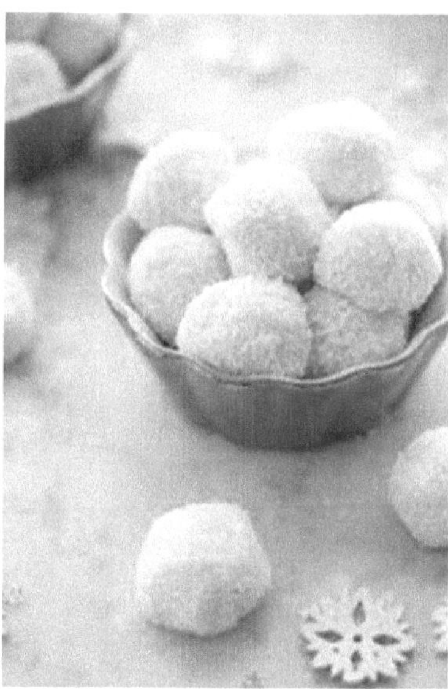

Serving: 12 fat bombs

Prep Time: 3 hours

Cook Time: 5 minutes

Ingredients

*   12 drops of liquid stevia

*   1 tsp of shredded coconut, unsweetened

*   1⁄4 cup of coconut oil

*   1⁄4 cup of cocoa butter

*   1 tsp of vanilla extract

Instructions

*   Combine cocoa butter, coconut oil, vanilla, and the stevia in some small saucepan placed over medium heat, while stirring frequently until the ingredients have melted, then turn off heat.

*   Add coconut then stir well so as to combine.

*   Pour your mixture into the 12 molds of silicone-bottomed ice cube tray or the silicone candy mold tray to be 3⁄4 full.

*   Freeze until it's set. Serve from a freezer.

Nutrients per one serving: Calories: 82, Fat: 9g, Protein: 0g, Sodium: 0mg, Fiber: 0g, Carbohydrates: 0g, Sugar: 0g

Almond Cookie Popsicles

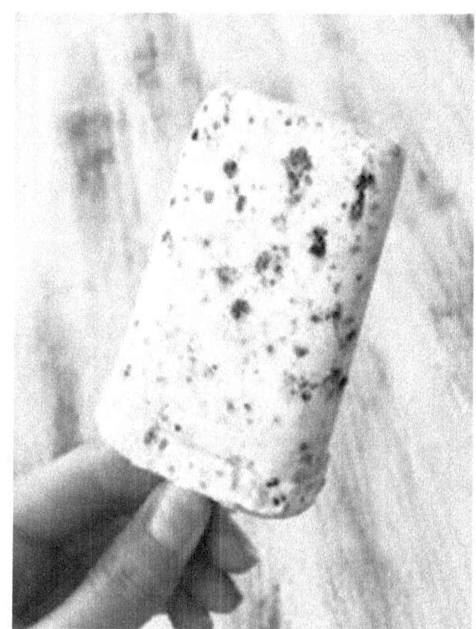

Serving: 8 fat bombs

Prep Time: 8–12 hours

Cook Time: 0 minutes

Ingredients

- 1 teaspoon of vanilla extract

- 1/4 cup of erythritol

- 1 1/2 cups of coconut cream, chilled

- 1/2 cup of almond butter

Instructions

- Put all your ingredients in some blender then blend until they are mixed completely, about 30 seconds.

- Pour the mix into the 8 Popsicle molds, while tapping the molds so as to dislodge the air bubbles.

- Freeze for about 8 hours.

•   Remove the popsicles from the molds. If the popsicles become hard to be removed from the containers, run the molds under the hot water briefly then the popsicles will become loose.

Nutrients per one serving: Calories: 294, Fat: 17g, Protein: 5g, Sodium: 94mg, Fiber: 1g, Carbohydrates: 39g, Sugar: 30g

Mocha Ice Bombs

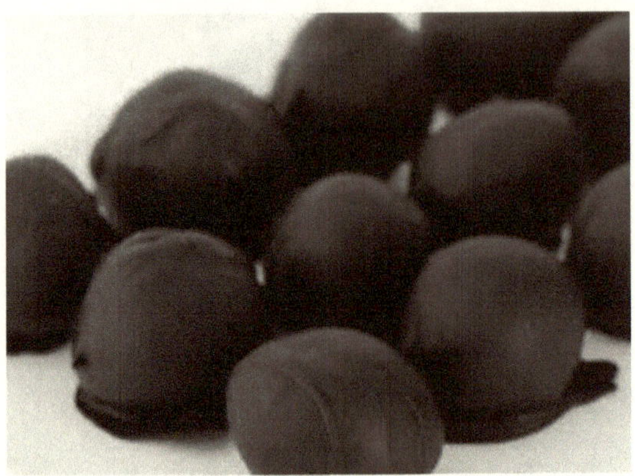

Serving: 12 people

Prep Time: 10 min

Ingredients

Mocha Ice Bombs

•   1/4cupof powdered sweetener

•   2 tbsp. of unsweetened cocoa

•   1/4cup of strong coffee chilled

•   1cup of cream cheese

Chocolate coating

•   70g of melted chocolate

•   28g of melted cocoa butter

Instructions

- Add coffee to cream cheese, the cocoa, and the sweetener.

- Blend until smooth.

- To make an ice bomb shape, just roll 2 tablespoons of mocha ice bomb mixture then place them on a tray or a plate lined with a baking parchment.

- Chocolate coating

- Mix your melted chocolate and the cocoa butter together.

- Roll every ice bomb in chocolate coating then place back on a lined tray/plate.

- Place in a freezer for about 2 hours.

Nutrients per one serving: Calories 127, Total fat 12.9g, Total Carbs 2.2g, Protein 1.9g

Butter Pecan Popsicles

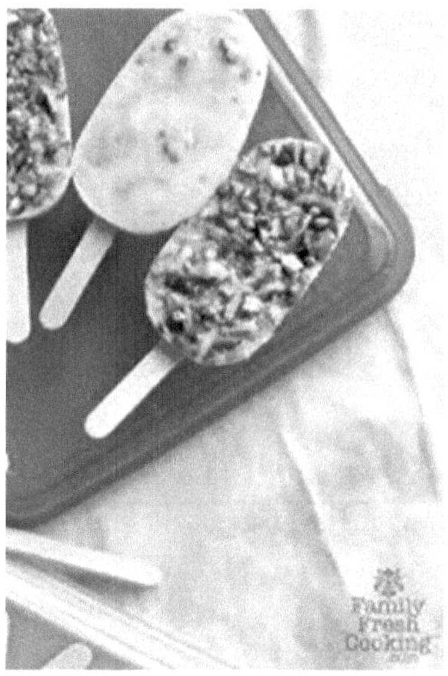

Serving: 8 fat bombs

Prep Time: 10 hours

Cook Time: 5 minutes

Ingredients

- 2 tablespoons of butter

- 1 1/2 cups of heavy cream

- 1 teaspoon of vanilla extract

- 1/8 teaspoon of salt

- 1 cup of coarsely chopped pecans

- 1 tablespoon of erythritol

Instructions

- In some medium nonstick pan placed over medium heat, just melt butter. Add pecans and a tablespoon of sweetener then cook for about 3 minutes, then keep aside to cool.

- In some blender, mix the cream, 2 tablespoons of sweetener, vanilla, and the salt for about 10 seconds.

- Scoop the cooled pecans into the bottom of the 8 Popsicle molds, while dividing them equally.

- Pour the cream mix into the molds, while tapping the molds so as to dislodge the air bubbles.

- Freeze for about 8 hours.

- Remove the popsicles from the molds. If the popsicles become hard to dislodge from the containers, just run the molds under the hot water and the popsicles will become loose.

Nutrients per one serving: Calories: 276, Fat: 29g Protein: 2g, Sodium: 54mg, Fiber: 1g, Carbohydrates: 8g, Sugar: 1g

Butter Rum Chocolate

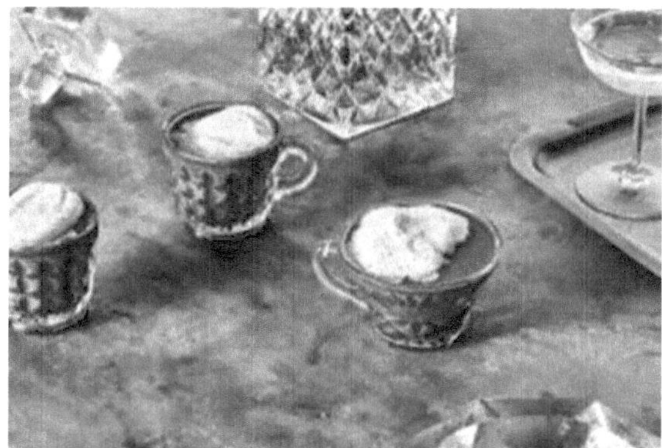

Serving: 12 fat bombs

Prep Time: 3 hours

Cook Time: 5 minutes

Ingredients

- 12 drops of liquid stevia

- 2 tablespoons of cocoa powder

- 1/4 cup of coconut oil

- 1/4 cup of almond butter

- 2 teaspoons of rum extract

Instructions

- Combine all the ingredients other than cocoa powder in some small saucepan placed over medium heat, while stirring frequently until the ingredients melt. Turn off heat.

- Add the cocoa powder then stir well so as to combine.

- Pour the mixture into 12 molds until each is about 3/4 full.

- Freeze until set then serves from the freezer.

Nutrients per one serving: Calories: 75, Fat: 7g, Protein: 2g, Sodium: 25mg, Fiber: 1g, Carbohydrates: 2g, Sugar: 1g

Strawberry

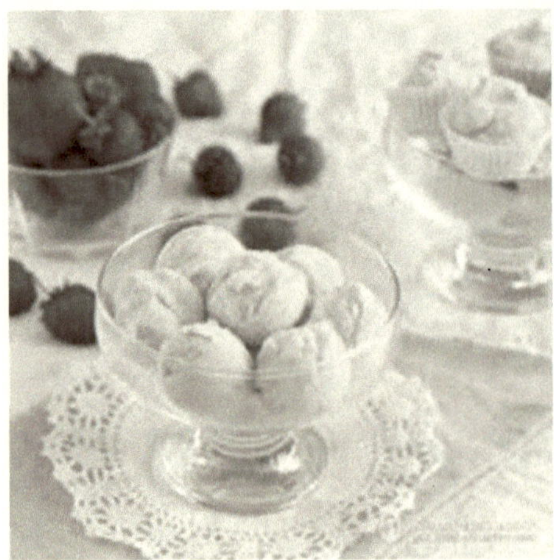

Serving: 6 people

Prep Time: 1 hr. 30 min

Ingredients

- 4 tablespoons of butter

- 50 grams of strawberry diced

- 1/4 cup of sugar equivalent or 1 tbsp. + 2 tsp of Truvia

- 4 tablespoons of coconut oil

- 2 ounces of heavy cream

Instructions

- Dice the strawberries then add heavy cream.

- Blend them together using an immersion blender.

- Melt butter in the microwave for about 30 secs then set aside.

- Measure out the coconut oil then set aside. Avoid heating.

- Add sweetener then combine all the ingredients well with an immersion blender.

- With some piping bag, pipe the fat bombs into a mold or a spoon mixture.

- Freeze for at least 20 minutes.

- Remove the bunnies from the mold, the place on a wax paper and melt a piece or some less sugar-free chocolate.

- Using a toothpick, just dab on the eyes and the nose for real peep look. Put back in a freezer for other 10-20 minutes. Put in a freezer.

Nutrients per one serving: 1086 Calories, 122g Fat, 2g Protein, 5g Carbohydrate, 1g Dietary Fiber, 4 net carbs.

Hazelnut Cappuccino Popsicles

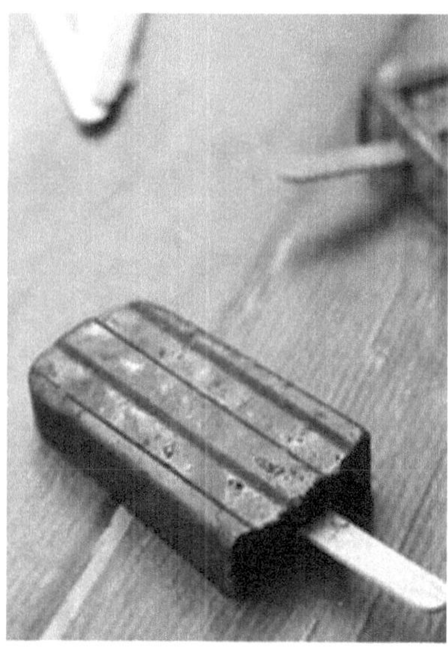

Serving: 8 fat bombs

Prep Time: 10 hours

Cook Time: 1 min

Ingredients

- 1 cup of espresso or strong coffee

- 1/4 cup of erythritol or granular Swerve

- 1/2 cup of crumbled hazelnuts

- 1 cup of heavy whipping cream

- 1/8 teaspoon of hazelnut flavor

Instructions

- Place all the ingredients other than hazelnuts in some blender then blend until mixed, for about 30 seconds.

- Pour the mixture into 8 Popsicle molds, while tapping molds so as to dislodge the air bubbles.

- Freeze for 8 hours.

- In some small nonstick pan placed over medium heat, just toast the crumbled hazelnuts for about 1 minute, while stirring constantly.

- Remove the popsicles from the molds. In case the popsicles become hard to be removed from the containers, just run molds under the hot water for the popsicles to become loose.

- Before you can serve, press the popsicles into the hazelnut crumbles so that they can coat on the outside.

Nutrients per one serving: Calories: 148, Fat: 15g, Protein: 2g, Sodium: 11mg, Fiber: 1g, Carbohydrates: 8g, Sugar: 0g

Coconut Vanilla Popsicles

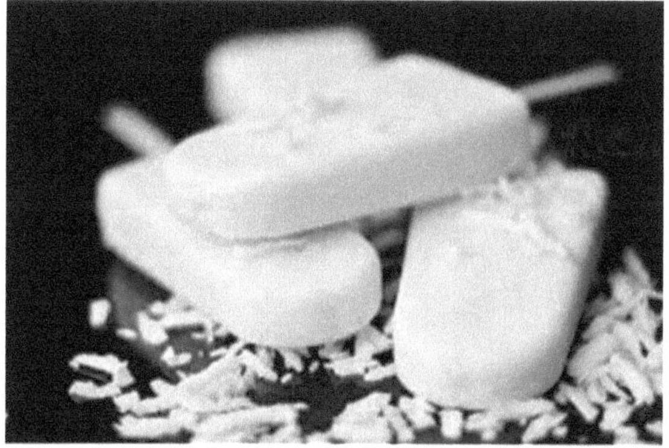

Serving: 8 fat bombs

Prep Time: 10 hours

Ingredients

*   2 cups of coconut cream, chilled

*   1/4 cup of unsweetened shredded coconut

*   1 teaspoon of vanilla extract

*   1/4 cup of erythritol or a granular Swerve

Instructions

*   Place your ingredients in some blender then blend until they are mixed completely, for about 30 seconds.

*   Pour the mix into your 8 Popsicle molds, while tapping molds so as to dislodge the air bubbles.

*   Freeze for about 8 hours.

*   Remove the popsicles from your molds. If the popsicles become hard to be removed from the containers, just run the molds under hot water for the popsicles to become loose.

Nutrients per one serving: Calories: 274, Fat: 13g, Protein: 1g, Sodium:

27mg, Fiber: 0g, Carbohydrates: 46g, Sugar: 38g

Easy Pumpkin Fat Bombs

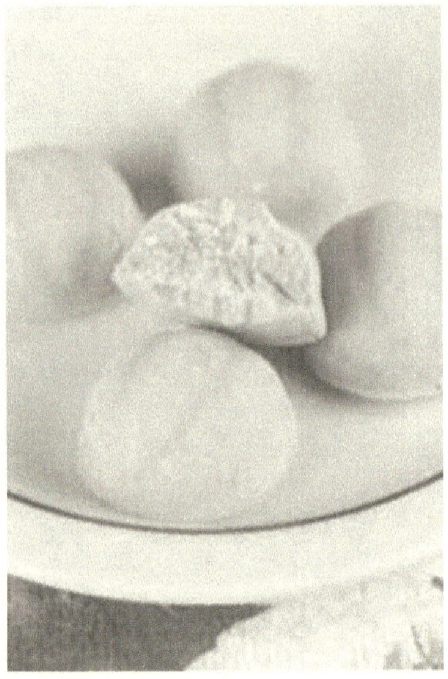

Ingredients

- 1/2 cup butter

- 10 drops liquid Stevia

- 1 tablespoon pumpkin spice extract

- 1 cup pure pumpkin puree

- 1 pound of softened cream cheese

Instructions

• Remove the cream cheese and the butter from the package and put them in a mixing bowl. Place at room temperature for 1 hour.

• Once the butter and the cream cheese have become soft, add pumpkin puree to butter and the cream cheese then blend together using some hand mixer or a whisk until it becomes smooth and combined.

• Add liquid Stevia and the pumpkin spice extract then continue blending for 30 seconds.

• Spoon evenly into the ice cube trays, then cover and put in a freezer for about 2 – 3 hours.

Nutrients per one serving: Calories: 89, Carbs: 1.3g, Fiber: 0.4g, Net Carbs: 0.9g, Fat: 8.3g, Protein: 1.3g, Vitamin A: 27.1%, Vitamin C: 0.1%, Calcium: 1.3%, Iron: 0.3%

Ginger Cream Popsicles

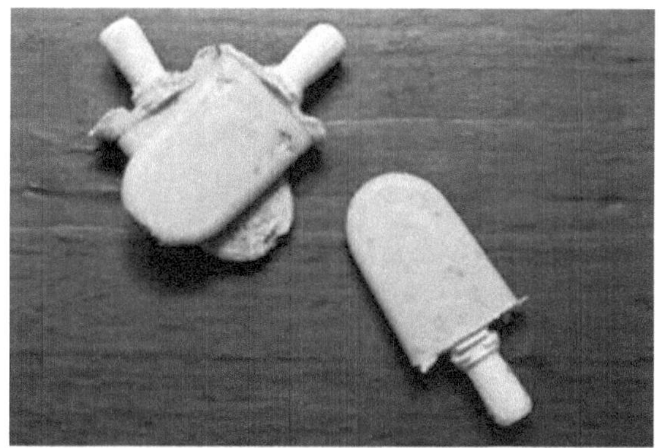

Serving: 8 fat bombs

Prep Time: 10 hours

Ingredients

• 2 cups of chilled coconut cream

• 2 tablespoons of coconut oil

• 1 teaspoon of ground ginger

• 1/4 cup of erythritol or granular Swerve

Instructions

• Place all the ingredients in a blender then blend until mixed completely, for about 30 seconds.

• Pour the mixture into 8 Popsicle molds, while tapping the molds so as to dislodge the air bubbles.

• Freeze for about 8 hours.

• Remove the popsicles from the molds. In case the popsicles become hard to be removed from the containers, just run molds under the hot water for the popsicles to become loose.

Nutrients per one serving: Calories: 295, Fat: 15g, Protein: 1g, Sodium: 27mg, Fiber: 0g, Carbohydrates: 46g, Sugar: 38g

Low Carb Frozen Chocolate Chip Balls

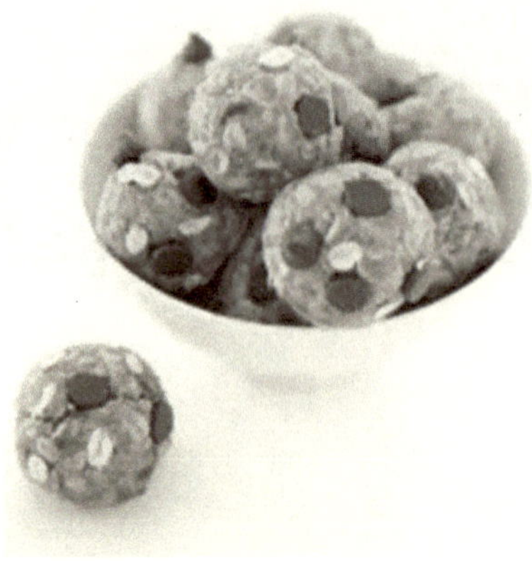

Serving: 16 people

Prep Time: 10 min

Ingredients

• 1/4 cup of cocoa powder, unsweetened

• 1/2 cup of Splenda (granulated)

• 1/2 cup of low carb chocolate chips

• 1/4 cup of water

- 1 Brick of cream cheese

- 1 stick of unsalted butter

Instructions

- Mix the cocoa powder and the water until some thick paste is formed.

- Add the cream cheese, butter, cocoa mixture, and Splenda to some stand mixer then blend until smooth.

- Stir in chocolate chips.

- Form your mixture into 16 balls of 1" diameter. Put on some tray or a pan lined with a silicone mat or a baking parchment.

- Freeze for 1 hour then transfer to a lidded container.

- Remove from freezer about 10 minutes before you can eat.

Nutrients per one serving: Total carbs 5.7g, Fiber 06g, Protein 3.6g, Fat 34.6g, Magnesium 15mg, Potassium 94mg

Chocolate Peanut Butter Cheesecake Bombs

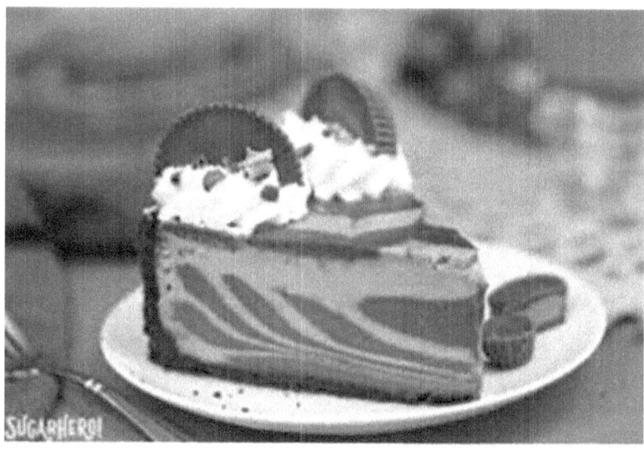

Serving: 12 people

Prep Time: 1 hr.

Ingredients

- 6 oz. of Cream Cheese

- 1/3 cup of Natural Creamy Peanut Butter

- 2 tbsps. of Xylitol

- 1 tsp of Vanilla Extract

- 1 pinch of

- 1 cup of Heavy Cream

- 1/8 tbsp. of Xanthan Gum

- 3 bars of Double Chocolate Crunch Bar, Snack Caramel

Instructions

- Beat the softened cream cheese using a mixer placed on medium speed to become creamy. Add powdered granular sugar substitute, peanut butter, and vanilla then beat to combine. Taste then increase the sweetness if needed by adding some pinch of stevia.

- Add 1 cup of cream and the 1/4 teaspoon of xanthan gum, beating until it becomes light and fluffy.

- Cut the Atkins bars lengthwise to form three segments and finely chop segments. Fold into the mixture. By use of a 2 tablespoon scoop onto wax paper readily covered with a baking sheet.

- Put in a freezer until frozen.

Nutrients per one serving: Calories 208, Protein 5.2g, Fiber 5.3g, Fat 18.3g

Peanut Butter Balls

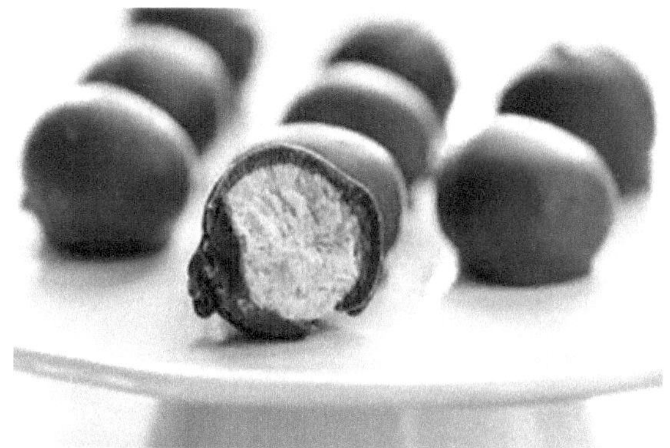

Serving: 15 balls

Prep Time: 10 min

Cook Time: 15 min

Ingredients

*   1 cup of Peanut Butter

*   3 oz. of Bakers Chocolate

*   1 cup of Almond Flour

*   1/4 cup of erythritol/swerve confectioner

Instructions

*   Combine almond flour, peanut butter and sweetener then combine well.

*   Place the peanut butter mixture into a freezer for 1 hour.

*   Melt the bakers chocolate in a microwave or a double boiler.

*   Roll the peanut butter mixture (frozen) into balls.

*   Insert a toothpick into the balls then coat in the melted chocolate.

*   Place the peanut butter balls coated with chocolate into the fridge so

as to harden, then store in the fridge.

Nutrients per one serving: Calories: 180, Fat: 15.1g, Carbs: 6.9g, Fiber: 3.6g, Protein: 7.2g, NET CARBS: 3.3g

Ultimate Keto Ice-Cream

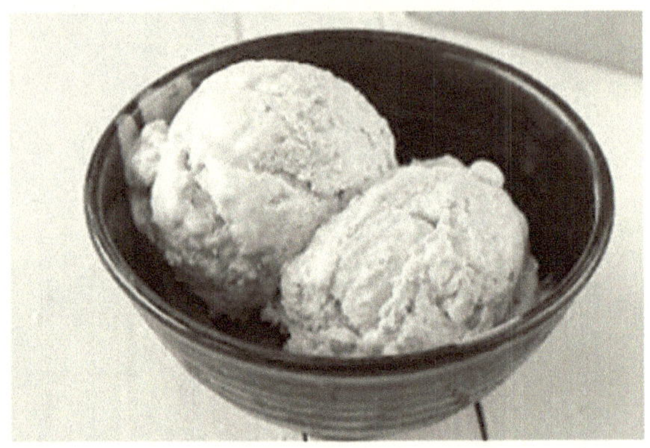

Serving: 8 people

Prep Time: 1 hr.

Ingredients

- ¼ cup of Erythritol

- 25-30 drops of Stevia extract

- 1 cup of coconut milk

- ½ cup of extra virgin coconut oil

- ½ cup of butter

- 4 large of egg yolks

- 2 large of eggs

- 2 vanilla beans

Instructions

- Separate egg yolks from the egg whites. Ensure butter and the coconut oil have been softened at room temperature.

•   Mix the coconut oil, butter, vanilla extract, the powdered Erythritol, and the stevia together.

•   Slowly add egg yolks and the whole eggs as you blend one by one then process until they are smooth.

•   Pour in coconut milk then continue blending.

•   Scoop your mixture into ice-cream maker then process depending on manufacturer's instructions.

•   Remove from ice-cream maker when half-way made. Use immersion blender then pulse until smooth.

•   Return to the ice-cream maker and continue until your ice-cream is done. If you see lumps, pulse by use of an immersion blender. Eat immediately or just place in a freezer for 30-60 minutes. Enjoy!

Nutrients per one serving: Total carbs 2.3g, Fiber 06g, Protein 3.6g, Fat 34.6g, Magnesium 15mg, Potassium 94mg

Creamy Peanut Butter Popsicles

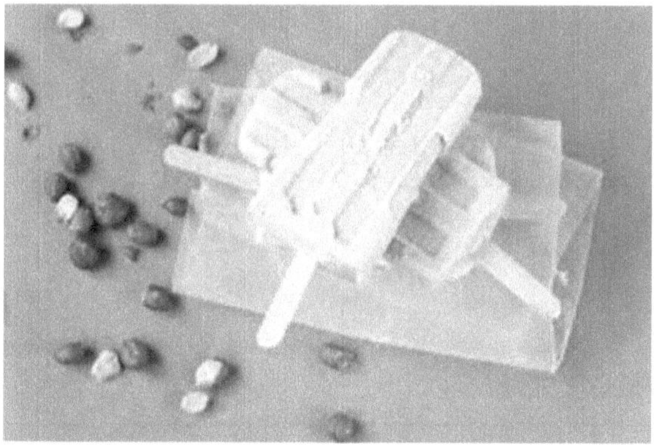

Serving: 8 fat bombs

Prep Time: 10 hours

Cook Time: 8 minutes

Ingredients

- 1 teaspoon of vanilla extract

- 1 ounce of unsweetened baking chocolate

- 1 tablespoon of confectioners Swerve

- 1/2 cup of mascarpone

- 1/2 cup of unsweetened peanut butter

- 1 Cup of heavy cream

- 1 tablespoon of erythritol or granular Swerve

Instructions

- In some small saucepan placed over low heat, just combine peanut butter, mascarpone, and cream. Stir well until melted, for about 3 minutes. Keep aside to cool.

- In some blender, add the cream mixture, the sweetener, and the vanilla. Blend well until combined, for about 10 seconds.

- Pour the cream mixture into your molds, while tapping the molds so as to dislodge the air bubbles.

- Freeze for at least 8 hours.

- In some double boiler placed over medium-low heat, just melt the chocolate and the confectioners Swerve.

- Remove the popsicles from your molds. If the popsicles become hard to be removed from containers, just run molds under the hot water briefly and the popsicles will become loose.

- Use a spoon to drizzle the melted chocolate each Popsicle then serve immediately.

Nutrients per one serving: Calories: 288, Fat: 28g, Protein: 6g, Sodium: 134mg, Fiber: 2g, Carbohydrates: 11g, Sugar: 3g

Matcha Popsicles

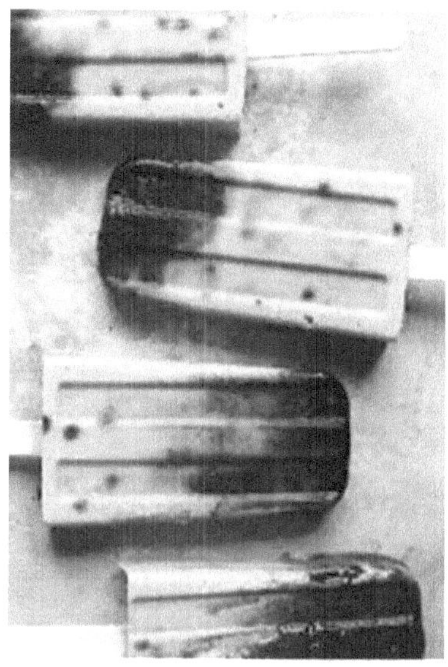

Serving: 8 people

Prep Time: 10 hours

Ingredients

- 1 teaspoon of matcha

- 1/4 cup of erythritol or granular Swerve

- 2 cups of chilled coconut cream

- 2 tablespoons of coconut oil

Instructions

- Place all the ingredients in your blender then blend until mixed completely, for about 30 seconds.

- Pour the mixture into 8 the Popsicle molds, while tapping the molds so as to dislodge the air bubbles.

- Freeze for 8 hours.

- Remove the popsicles from the molds. In case the popsicles become hard to be removed from the containers, just run molds under the hot water for the popsicles to become loose.

Nutrients per one serving: Calories: 294, Fat: 15g, Protein: 1g, Sodium: 88mg, Fiber: 0g, Carbohydrates: 46g, Sugar: 38g

Valentine's Day Keto Fat Bombs

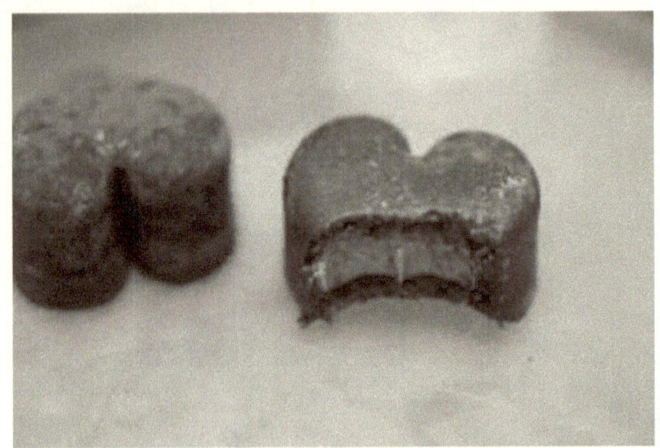

Serving: 4 people

Prep time: 2 min

Cook time: 2 min

Ingredients

- 1 teaspoon of Cocoa Powder

- 2 Oz of Dark Chocolate

- 8 Drops of EZ-Sweetz

- 2 Oz. of Almond Butter

- 2 Oz. of Coconut Oil

- 1 Oz. of Cream Cheese

- ½ Oz. of Torani Sugar-Free Vanilla Syrup

Instructions

- Combine all items other than almond butter then microwave for about 30 seconds

- Stir in ingredients and microwave again then keep on stirring if the chocolate fails to melt.

- Pour the base layer into the mold you are using

- Then by use of a spoon, place some dollop of the Almond Butter at the center.

- Fill in the remaining mold to the top

- Freeze until your chocolate becomes hard, then hard push these out of the mold

- Store in a fridge

Nutrients per one serving: Calories 297, Fat 30, Carbs 7, Fiber 3, Protein 5

Orange Chocolate Popsicles

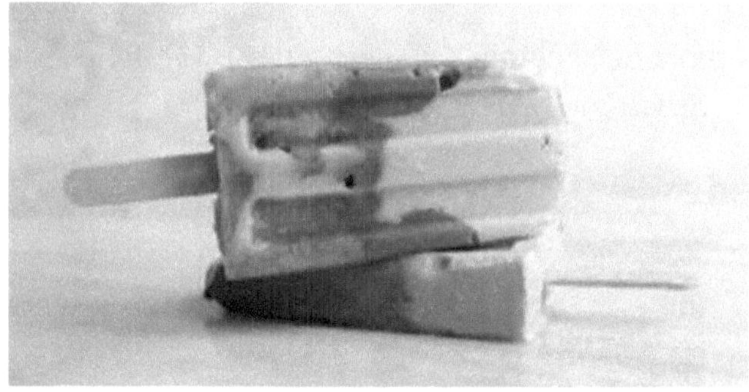

Serving: 4 fat bombs

Prep Time: 10 hours

Ingredients

- 1 teaspoon of orange zest

- 1 medium pitted and peeled avocado

- 1/8 teaspoon of orange extract

- 1/8 teaspoon of salt

- 1/2 cup of coconut cream

- 1/2 cup of cocoa powder

- 1 tablespoon of erythritol or granular Swerve

Instructions

- Place all the ingredients in some small food processor or a blender then blend until mixed completely, for about 30 seconds.

- Pour the mixture into 4 Popsicle molds, while tapping the molds so as to dislodge the air bubbles.

- Freeze for 8 hours or overnight.

- Remove the popsicles from the molds. In case the popsicles become hard to be removed from the containers, just run molds under the hot water for the popsicles to become loose.

Nutrients per one serving: Calories: 237, Fat: 15g, Protein: 4g, Sodium: 93mg, Fiber: 7g, Carbohydrates: 36g, Sugar: 20g

Ice Cream

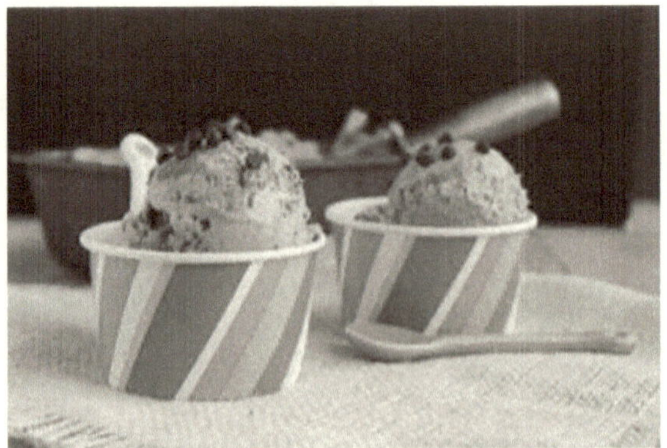

Serving: 5 people

Prep Time: 10 min

Ingredients

*   1/3 cup of xylitol

*   1/3 cup of flavor variation

*   ¼ cup of MCT oil

*   4 pastured eggs, whole

*   4 yolks of pastured eggs

*   1/3 cup of melted cacao butter

*   1/3 cup of melted coconut oil

*   2 tsp of vanilla bean powder

*   8-10 ice cubes

Instructions

*   Add all the ingredients other than the ice cubes into a jug of a high powdered blender. Blend this on high for about 2 minutes, or until creamy.

*   As the blender runs, remove the top portion of the lid then drop in an ice cube, one at a time, while allowing your blender to run for about 10 seconds between every ice cube.

*   Once you have added all ice, pour your cold mixture into the ice cream maker then churn it on high for about 20-30 minutes, based on the ice cream maker.

*   Serve this immediately as a soft-serve or scoop it into 9 * 5 loaf pan then freeze for about 45 minutes. Store while covered in freezer for about a week.

Nutrients per one serving: Calories: 431, Calories from Fat: 399, Saturated Fat: 34 g, Total Fat: 44.3, Sodium: 56 mg, Carbs: 3.4 g,

Cholesterol: 299> mg, Dietary Fiber: 1.6 g, Protein: 7.7 g, Net Carbs: 1.8 g

Dark Chocolate Popsicles

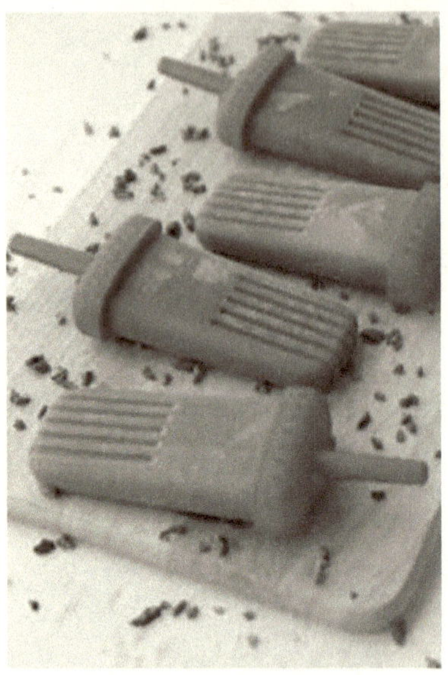

Serving: 4 fat bombs

Prep Time: 10 hours

Ingredients

- 1 medium pitted and peeled avocado

- 1/8 teaspoon of vanilla extract

- 1/2 cup of coconut cream

- 1/3 cup of cocoa powder

- 1 tablespoon of erythritol

- 1/8 teaspoon of salt

Instructions

- Place your ingredients in some small food processor or a blender then blend until mixed completely, for about 30 seconds.

• Pour the mixture into 4 Popsicle molds, while tapping the molds so as to dislodge the air bubbles.

• Freeze for about 8 hours.

• Remove the popsicles from molds. In case the popsicles become hard to be removed from the containers, just run molds under the hot water for the popsicles to become loose.

Nutrients per one serving: Calories: 229, Fat: 14g, Protein: 3g, Sodium: 92mg, Fiber: 6g, Carbohydrates: 37g, Sugar: 20g

Mint Chocolate Chip Popsicles

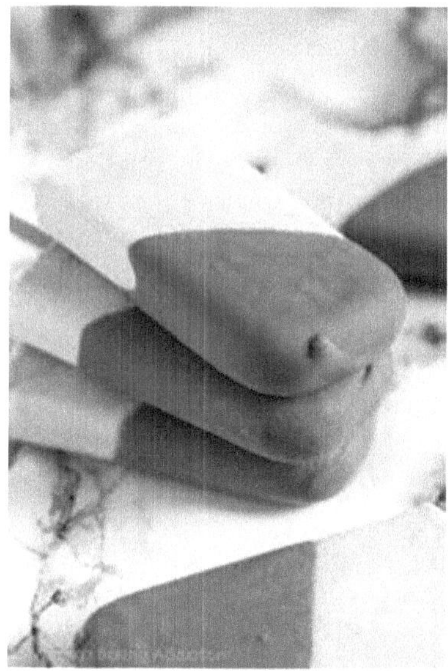

Serving: 8 fat bombs

Prep Time: 10 hours

Cook Time: 5 min

Ingredients

1 ounce of unsweetened chocolate chips

1/4 cup of erythritol or granular Swerve

2 cups of coconut cream

1 cup of fresh mint leaves

Instructions

•	Combine the coconut milk and the mint in some medium saucepan placed over medium heat.

•	Simmer until some bubbles begin to appear, for about 5 minutes.

•	Remove from the heat then allow to steep for 20 minutes.

•	Strain through some fine-mesh sieve into a bowl.

•	Add the chocolate and the sweetener then stirs well.

•	Pour the mixture into 4 Popsicle molds, while tapping the molds so as to dislodge the air bubbles.

•	Freeze for 8 hours or overnight.

•	Remove the popsicles from the molds. In case the popsicles become hard to be removed from the containers, just run molds under the hot water for the popsicles to become loose.

Nutrients per one serving: Calories: 304, Fat: 16g, Protein: 2g, Sodium: 32mg, Fiber: 2g, Carbohydrates: 48g, Sugar: 38g

Raspberry Cheesecake Fat Bombs

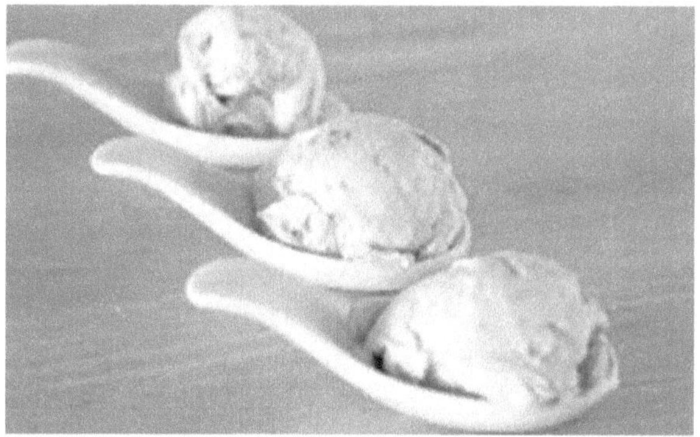

Serving: 16 people

Prep Time: 15 min

Cook Time: 1hr 15min

Ingredients

- 1 teaspoon of vanilla extract

- 2 tbsps. of Erythritol

- ½ cup of almond flour

- ¼ cup of coconut flour

- 250g of mascarpone

- 1 cup of raspberries

- 15-20 drops of liquid stevia (optional)

Coating:

- 80g of extra dark chocolate

- 40g of cacao butter

Instructions

• Put the mascarpone, frozen raspberries, Erythritol, and vanilla into your food processor then pulse until they are creamy and smooth.

• Add almond and the coconut flour then pulse again just so as to mix up. Spoon 2 tablespoons of your mixture into an ice tray that is good for creating fat bomb shapes. Put in freezer for about 45-60 minutes.

• Meanwhile, melt dark chocolate and the cacao butter in some double boiler or glass bowl on the top of some small saucepan readily filled with a cup of water over medium heat. Once melted completely, remove from heat then set aside for it to cool down.

• Remove your mixture from freezer. Pick one fat bomb each time then hold over your bowl with melted chocolate.

• Spoon chocolate over fat bomb until it is well-coated. Keep turning it until your chocolate becomes solidified. Put each coated fat bombs on the tray lined with a greaseproof paper then place in a fridge for about 15 minutes before you can serve.

• Keep in fridge for about one week or freeze for 3 months.

Nutrients per one serving: Total Carbs 3.1g, Fiber 1.2g, Protein 2.5g, Fat 12.8g, Magnesium 23mg, Potassium 78g

Spiced Cocoa Coolers

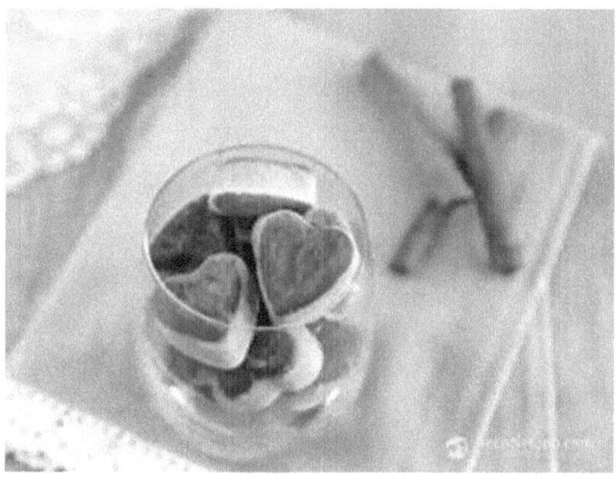

Serving: 10 people

Prep Time 1hr 30 min

Ingredients

- 1 cup of heavy whipping cream

- ¼ tsp of cayenne pepper

- 2 tbsps. of Erythritol

- 15-20 drops of Stevia extract

- 2 tbsps. of unsweetened cocoa powder

- 1 vanilla bean

- 1 tsp of cinnamon

Instructions

- Your ingredients will dissolve easily after warming up cream or the coconut milk slightly.

- Place all other ingredients in cream then mix until combined well.

- Pour your liquid into the ice-cube tray then transfer this into freezer for 1-2 hours. Enjoy!

Nutrients per one serving: Total carbs 1.8g, Fiber 0.7g, Protein 0.7g, Fat 5g

Blueberry Cheesecake Popsicles

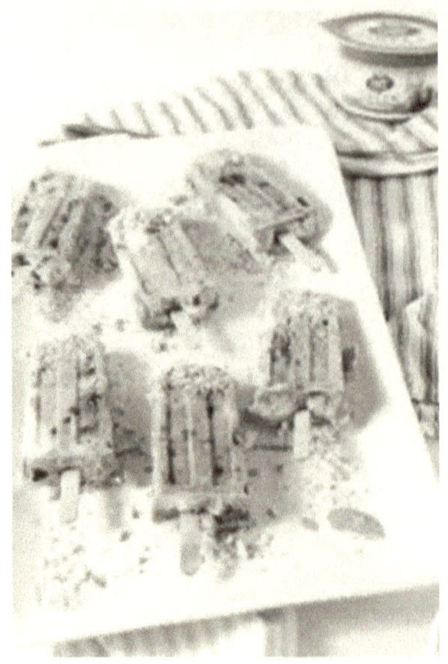

Serving: 10 people

Prep Time: 5 minutes

Ingredients

*   8 Tbsps. of light cream cheese

*   6 Tbsps. of icing sugar

*   2 cups of fresh blueberries

*   30 Tbsps. of Cool Whip

Instructions

*   Puree the blueberries and cream cheese and the icing sugar in your blender until smooth.

*   Fold in the whipped topping gently.

- Spoon into the popsicle molds then freeze until firm.

- Run the mold under some hot water so as to loosen the popsicles so that they become easy to unmold.

Nutrients per one serving: 83 calories, 3 fat, 1 protein, 15 carbs.

Blueberry Fat Bombs

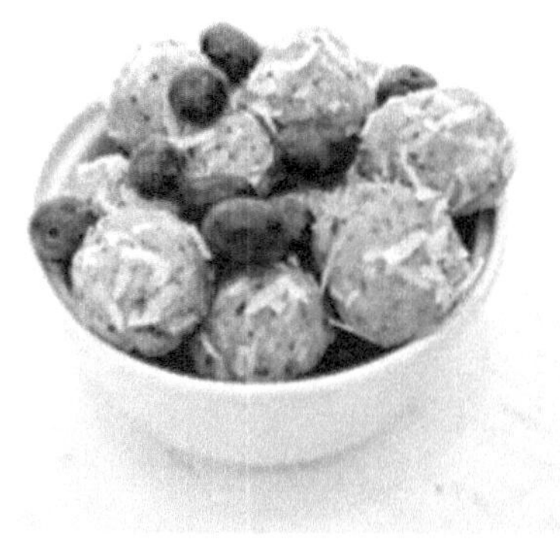

Serving: 24 fat bombs

Prep Time: 10 min

Ingredients

- 1 stick of butter (4 oz.)

- Scant cup of blueberries

- 3/4 c. of coconut oil

- 4 oz. of softened cream cheese

- ¼ c. of coconut cream

- Sweetener to taste

Instructions

- In a food processor, place the coconut cream, berries, and soft cream cheese.

- Puree until it is smooth.

- Over low heat in a saucepan, melt coconut oil and butter.

- Let cool for about 5 minutes and then add to the food processor then puree again until it is smooth.

- Slowly, add any sweetener of your choice while tasting and adjusting it to your liking.

- Transfer the mixture into molds. Leave space at the top.

- Freeze in a freezer for one hour and then enjoy.

- You can also freeze them in suitable plastic bags.

Nutrients per one serving: 116 calories, 44g protein, 13g fat, 1.02g carbs 84g NET CARBS, .18g fiber.

SWEET FAT BOMBS RECIPES

Cream Cheese Fat Bombs

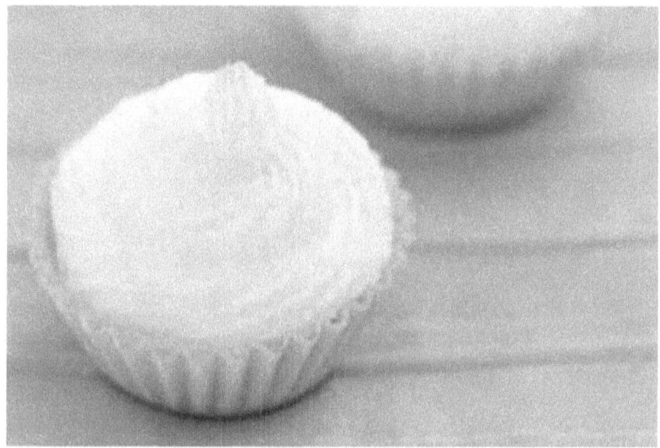

Serving: 2 balls

Prep Time: 10 minutes

Cook Time: 5 minutes

Ingredients

- Sugar free jello, 1 package, or pudding mix

- 1 8oz package Kraft Philadelphia cream cheese

Instructions

- Take a package of Cream cheese then cut it into 16 squares.

- Put jello or the pudding mix into a small bowl.

- Take each square then cover using a pudding mix on all the sides.

- Roll into some ball in hands.

- Keep covered with a plastic wrap inside your fridge.

Nutrients per one serving: 105 calories, 9 g fat, 1 carb, and 3 g protein

Coconut Almond Butter Cups

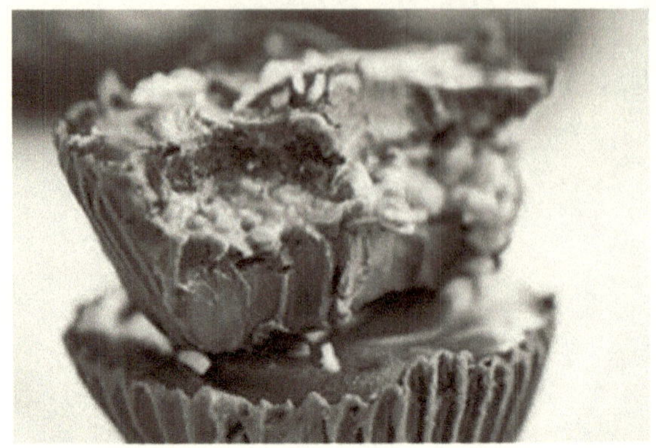

Serving: 12 cups

Prep Time: 5 minutes

Cook Time: 10 minutes

Ingredients

Bottom Layer:

- ½ cup of finely chopped cacao paste

- ¼ cup of coconut oil

- 1 tsp of vanilla powder

- ¼ tsp of ground Ceylon cinnamon

- 2-3 drops of pure almond extract

Middle Layer:

- ½ cup of almond butter, all natural

- ¼ cup of coconut oil

- ¼ tsp of ground Ceylon cinnamon

Top Layer:

- ¼ cup of coconut oil

- ½ cup of creamy coconut butter

Garnish:

Whole raw almonds

Toasted coconut flakes

Instructions

- Line muffin pan with parchment paper cups.

- Melt ¾ cup of coconut oil using one of your preferred methods.

- In some small mixing bowl, melt cacao paste in a microwave in intervals of 20-30 seconds while stirring well. Mix them delicately until they are combined completely.

- Divide melted chocolate between your 12 muffin cups then place in a fridge to set it for 5 minutes.

- Meanwhile, take some other mixing bowl, then add ground cinnamon, almond butter and ¼ cup of melted coconut oil.

- Stir well to combine, and pour this mixture evenly over your set chocolate. Put cups back to your fridge until a new layer has been set, for 5 to 10 minutes.

- As the cups are firming up, just add a ½ cup of the creamy coconut butter to your bowl which you had melted the coconut oil in then stir well until incorporated.

- Spoon the mixture over almond butter layer and garnish every cup with whole almond or pinch of some toasted coconut flakes.

- Put back to your refrigerator so as to finish setting for about 1 hour.

Nutrients per one serving: Calories 298, Total Fat 29.5g, Saturated fat 20.6g, Cholesterol 0mg, Sodium 6mg, Potassium 83mg, Total Carbohydrate 6.5g, protein 6.5g

Keto caramel pudding

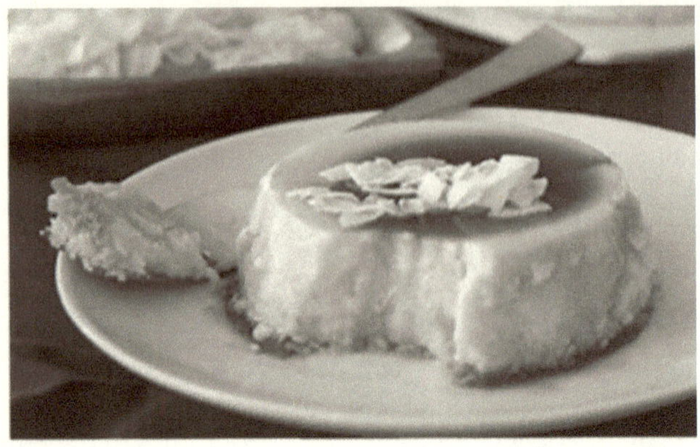

Servings 4

Total Time: 50 minutes + 8 hours for cooling

Ingredients:

- ¼ cup erythritol (for caramel sauce)

- ¼ cup erythritol (for cream)

- ⅛ cup water

- 1 cup fat cream

- 2 whole eggs

- 2 egg yolks

- 1 ½ tbsp butter

- 1 tbsp vanilla

Cooking process:

1.   In a saucepan, heat the erythritol to prepare the caramel. Add water and butter; stir until the sauce is golden. Pour sauce in ramekins.

2.   In a deep bowl, mix the cream, erythritol for cream and vanilla.

3.   In another bowl, beat the eggs and add the yolks. Mix again by a mixer.

4.   Add the egg mass into the creamy base. Mix to uniformity. Pour cream into the ramekins on the caramel layer.

5.   Put ramekins in a baking dish, filling it with half hot water.

6.   Bake in the oven at 175 °C for 35 minutes.

7.   To cool pudding and leave it in the refrigerator for 8-10 hours.

8.   Extract the contents of each ramekin on the dish bottom up.

Nutrients per one serving:

Calories: 297 | Fats: 31.4 g. | Carbohydrates: 2.3 g. | Proteins: 4.4 g.

Keto cottage cheese balls with chocolate glaze

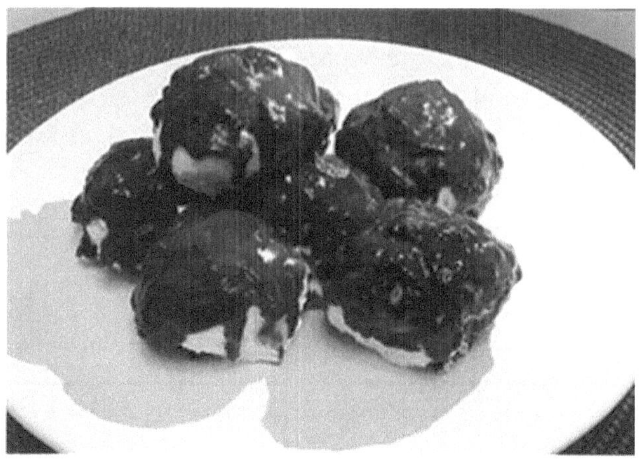

Servings 12

Total Time: 15 minutes + 40 minutes for freezing

Ingredients:

- 500 g fat cottage cheese

- 300 g coconut oil

- 2 tbsp sukrin

- 100 g dark chocolate

- 50 ml cream

Cooking process:

1. In a deep bowl, mix the cottage cheese with the sukrin. Add 200 g of coconut oil, and stir it until uniformity.

2. Form the small balls, lay out in a container and put in the freezer for 15 minutes.

3. In a water bath, melt the chopped chocolate. Add 100 g of coconut oil and cream. Stir mass and simmer for 5 minutes.

4. Pour cottage cheese balls with chocolate glaze and leave in the freezer for 25 minutes.

Nutrients per one serving:

Calories: 280 | Fats: 435 g. | Carbohydrates: 19 g. | Proteins: 80 g.

Chocolate Macadamia Fat Bomb

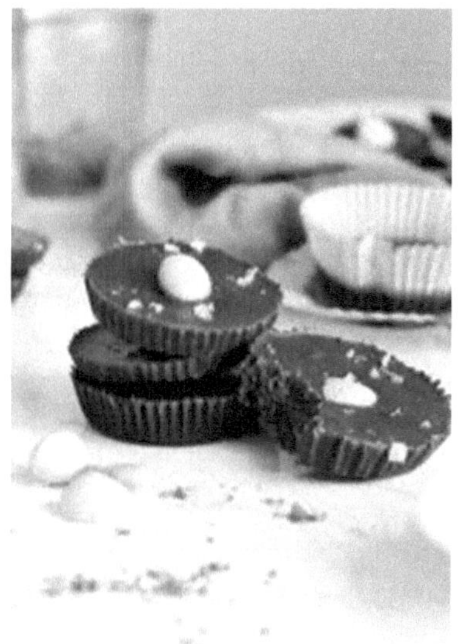

Serving: 6 people

Prep Time: 5 minutes

Cook Time: 5 minutes

Ingredients

- 4 oz. of Chopped macadamias

- ¼ cup of Heavy cream or the coconut oil

- 2 oz. of Cocoa Butter

- 2 Tbs of unsweetened cocoa powder

- 2 Tbs of Swerve

Instructions

- Melt the cocoa butter in some small saucepan in a bath of water.

- Put cocoa powder to a saucepan.

- Add Swerve then mix well until the ingredients are blended well and melted.

- Add the macadamias then stir in well.

- Add cream, then mix well, bring it back to temperature.

- Pour in the molds or the paper candy cups.

- Allow to cool, then place in a fridge so as to harden.

- Keeps this at room temperature.

Nutrients per one serving: Calories 267, Fat 28gm, Net carbs 3gm, Protein 3gm

Almond Pistachio Fat Bombs

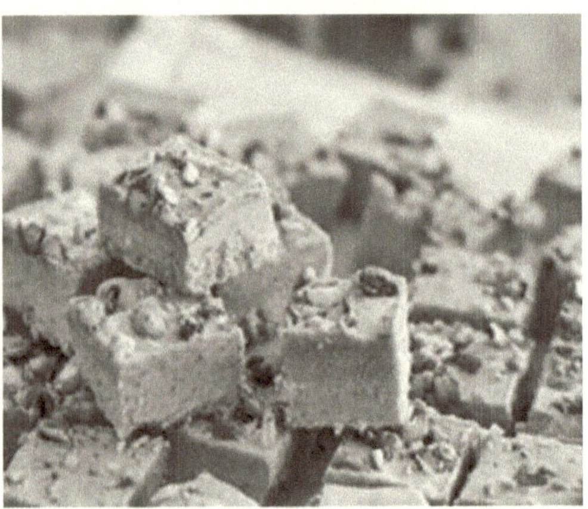

Serving: 36 squares

Prep Time: 5 minutes

Cook Time: 15 minutes

Ingredients

- ½ cup of melted and finely chopped cacao butter

- 1 cup of roasted almond butter, all natural

- 2 tsp of chai spice

- ¼ tsp of pure almond extract

- ¼ tsp of Himalayan Salt

- 1 cup of creamy coconut butter

- 1 cup of coconut oil

- ½ cup of coconut milk, full fat

- ¼ cup of ghee

- 1 tbsp. of pure vanilla extract

- ¼ cup of chopped raw shelled pistachios

Instructions

- Grease and line some 9" baking pan using a parchment paper, and leave some little bit hanging on the side for making unmolding easy. Set aside.

- Melt cacao butter in some small saucepan and set over a low heat or in a microwave, while stirring often. Reserve.

- Add all ingredients, except the cacao butter and the shelled pistachios, to some large mixing bowl. Just mix using a hand mixer, starting on low speed and then moving to a high speed until all your ingredients are combined well and your mixture becomes airy.

- Pour melted cacao butter into the almond mixture then resume mixing on a low speed until they are well incorporated.

- Transfer to a prepared pan then spread evenly and sprinkle using chopped pistachios.

- Refrigerate these until they are set completely.

- Cut so as to make 36 squares then splurge!

Nutrients per one serving: Calories 170, Total Fat 17.4g, Cholesterol

4mg, Sodium 18mg, Potassium 62mg, Total Carbohydrates 3.1g, Protein 2.2g

Toasted Coconut Fudge

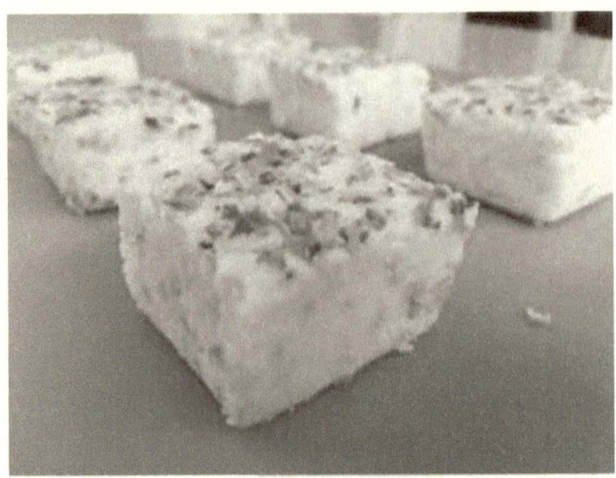

Serving: 36 squares

Prep Time: 10 minutes

Cook Time: 5 minutes

Ingredients

- ½ tsp of ground Ceylon cinnamon

- Few drops of pure almond extract

- ¼ cup of raw honey

- 6 cups of coconut flakes, organic toasted

- ½ cup of ghee

- ½ tsp of Himalayan salt

Instructions

- Grease some square pan with coconut oil then line it using parchment paper, and leave some bit of overhang at either end.

- Add some toasted coconut to a high-speed blender and then process on a medium speed for 30 seconds to 1 minute, and increase the speed slowly to the highest setting. Continue processing until your coconut flakes form a thick paste.

•	Remove your lid then scrape the sides using a rubber spatula, and add ghee, cinnamon, salt, and the almond extract. Begin processing, starting on a low and to the highest setting, until your mixture becomes smooth.

•	Add honey and start up the motor. Increase the speed to a medium-high then process until your honey becomes incorporated completely.

•	Transfer the mixture to a prepared pan then spread it evenly to the edge. Tap the sides gently for few times so as to remove potential air bubbles then make the top nice and smooth.

•	Place this in a cupboard so as to set until next day.

•	Run a spatula or knife around sides then gently pull on parchment paper so as to remove the fudge from your pan. Turn this upside down onto some cutting board then peel off parchment paper. Cut the fudge into 36 squares.

•	Keep this in a cool dry place, in some airtight container for a few months.

Nutrients per one serving: Calories 267, Fat 28gm, Net Carbs 3gm, Protein 3gm

Coconut Almond Butter Fat Bombs

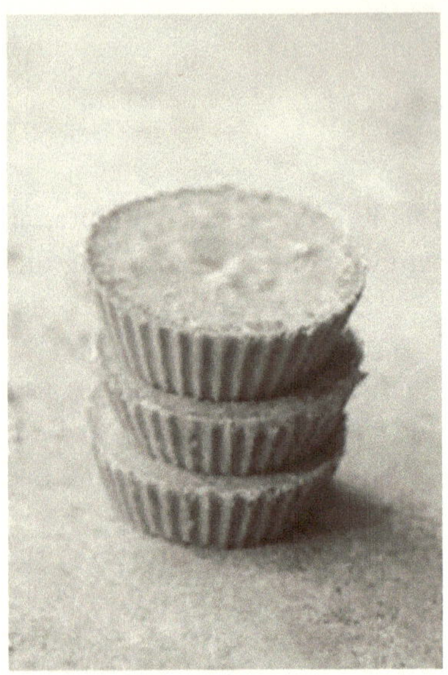

Serving: 24 people

Prep Time: 10 min

Cook Time: 20 min

Ingredients

- 3/4 cup of melted coconut oil

- 3 Tbs. of cocoa

- 9.5 Tbs. of almond butter

- 60 drops of liquid Stevia

- 9 Tbs. of melted salted butter

Instructions

- Pour scant 2 tablespoons into all the 24 candy or the mini muffin molds and then place the candy mold on a cookie sheet.

- Freeze for about 30 minutes, and pop out your Fat Bombs and keep them in some bag or any other container in your freezer.

Nutrients per one serving: 145 calories, 14.7g fat, 1.53g protein, 1.67g carbs

Low Carb Chocolate Coconut Fat Bombs

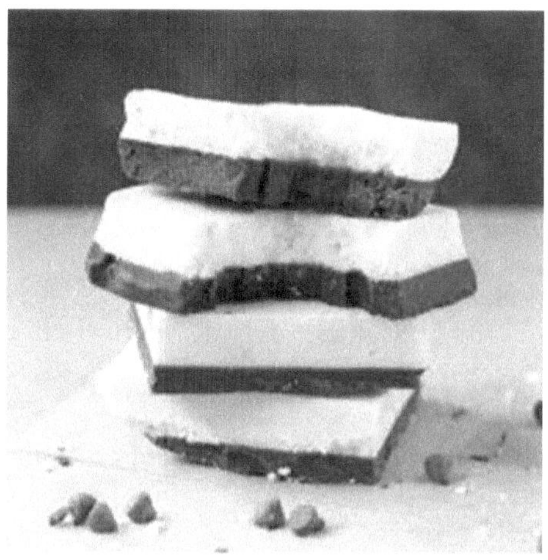

Serving: 10-12 balls

Prep time: 90 minutes

Cook time: 5 minutes

Ingredients

*   4 Tbsps. of quality cocoa powder

*   1 tsp of stevia powder extract

*   3-4 drops peppermint essential oil (optional)

*   1 cup of coconut butter

*   1 cup of coconut milk

*   1 tsp of vanilla extract

*   1 cup of coconut shreds

Instructions

- Place the glass bowl over saucepan having few inches of water so as to create some double boiler.

- Place all ingredients other than shredded coconut in the double boiler over a medium heat.

- Mix your ingredients as you wait for these to melt together.

- Once all ingredients are combined well, remove your bowl from heat.

- Place your bowl in a fridge until it becomes hard enough to be rolled into balls.

- Roll your contents into balls of one inch then roll them through coconut shreds.

- Place your balls on some plate and refrigerate for about one hour.

- Serve and enjoy.

Nutrients per one serving: Calories: 251, Total Fat: 21.7 g, Protein: 2.8 g, Total Carbs: 12.8 g, Fiber: 4.4 g Net Carbs: 8.4g

Easy Lemon Fat Bombs

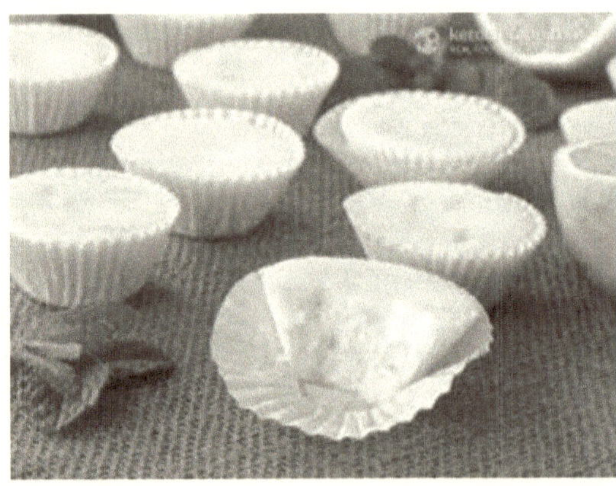

Serving: 16 people

Prep Time: 40-60 minutes

Ingredients

* Organic fresh lemon zest from 1-2 lemons

* 15-20 drops of Stevia extract

A pinch salt

* 7.1 oz of softened coconut butter

* ¼ cup of softened extra virgin coconut oil

Instructions

* Zest your lemons then ensure the coconut butter and the coconut oil have been softened.

* Mix all your ingredients in some bowl then make sure your lemon zest and the stevia have been distributed evenly. You may use lemon, clear or coconut stevia drops.

* Fill every silicone candy mold or mini muffin paper cup with ~ 1 tbsp. of coconut mixture then place it on some tray which can fit in your fridge.

* Place in your fridge for about 30-60 minutes.

* When done, put in a refrigerator. The coconut oil and the coconut butter will get soft while at room temperature.

Nutrients per one serving: Total Carbs 2.9g, Fiber 2.1g, Protein 0.76g, Fat 11.9g, Magnesium 5mg, Potassium 46mg

Chocolate Coconut Cups

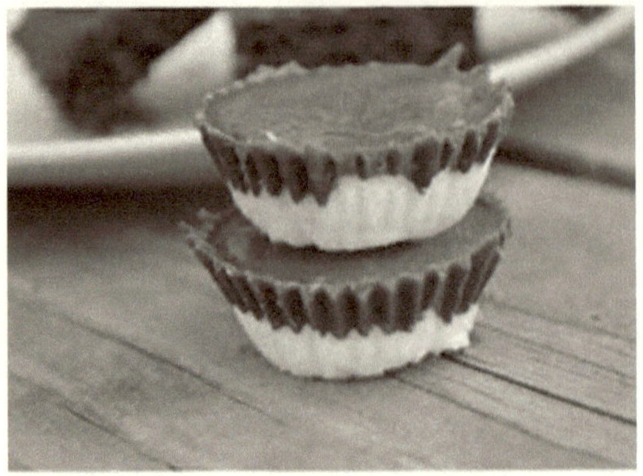

Serving: 20 mini-cups

Prep Time: 10 minutes

Cook Time: 10 minutes

Ingredients

Coconut Candies:

- 1/2 cup of coconut butter

- 1/2 cup of Kelapo coconut oil

- 1/2 cup of unsweetened shredded coconut

- 3 tbsps. of powdered Swerve Sweetener

Chocolate Topping:

- 1 & 1/2 ounces of Cocoa Butter

- 1 ounce of unsweetened chocolate

- 1/4 cup of powdered Swerve Sweetener

- 1/4 cup of cocoa powder

- 1/4 tsp of vanilla extract

Instructions

- For candies, line some mini-muffin pan using 20 mini paper liners.

- Combine the coconut butter and the coconut oil in some small saucepan over a low heat. Stir well until smooth and melted, then stir in the shredded coconut with the sweetener until combined.

- Divide the mixture amongst your prepared mini muffin cups then freeze until they are firm.

- For the chocolate coating, combine the cocoa butter and the unsweetened chocolate together in some bowl placed over a pan of some simmering water. Stir them well until they melt.

- Stir in sifted powdered sweetener, and stir in the cocoa powder, until it becomes smooth.

- Remove from the heat then stir in your vanilla extract.

- Spoon the chocolate topping over the chilled coconut candies then allow to set, for about 15 minutes.

- OR if you are using pre-packaged chocolate, just melt it and spoon over cold coconut filling.

- Candies can be kept on the countertop for about a week.

Nutrients per one serving: 5g of carbs, 4g of fiber, 25g Fat, 240 Calories, 2g Protein, 4g Dietary Fiber, 0mg Cholesterol, 5g Carbohydrate, 6mg Sodium.

Cocoa-Lemon Fat Bomb

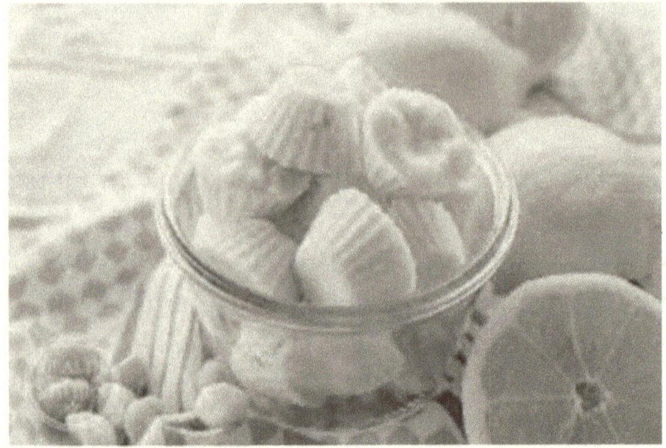

Serving: 24 people

Prep Time: 15 min

Ingredients

COATING:

- 4 oz. of edible cocoa butter

- ⅔ Cup of Swerve confectioners

- 1 tsp of lemon extract

- ¼ tsp of Celtic sea salt

FILLING:

- 1 cup of Swerve

- ½ cup of lemon juice

- 4 large eggs

- 1 tablespoon of lemon peel, finely grated

- 8 tablespoons of coconut oil

Instructions

• Put the cocoa butter in some double boiler then heat on medium high until it is fully melted.

• Stir in the natural sweetener.

• Stir in the extracts and salt.

• Place into a truffle mold then cool in a refrigerator until the white chocolate becomes solid.

• LEMON CURD FILLING: Mix the natural sweetener, 4 eggs, lemon juice and lemon peel in a medium saucepan then whisk so as to blend.

• Add the coconut oil. Whisk them constantly over medium heat until the mixture becomes thick and it coats back of your spoon thickly. Pour the mixture through a strainer into a medium bowl.

• Place the bowl in some larger bowl full of ice water then whisk it occasionally until the lemon curd becomes cooled completely.

Nutrients per one serving: 95 calories, 1.1g protein, 10.1g fat, 0.2g carbs

Happy Almond Bombs

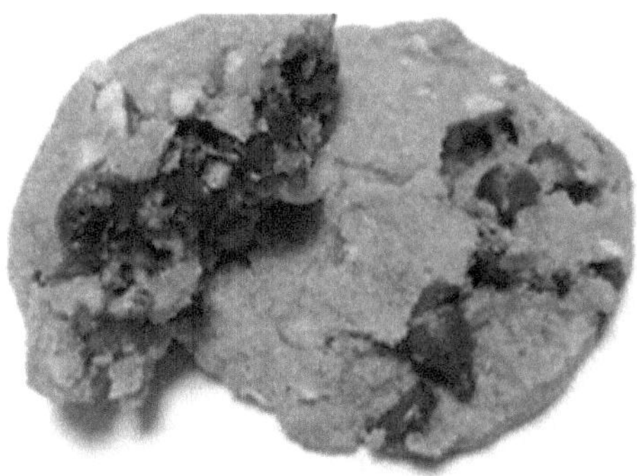

Serving: 4 people

Prep Time: 5 minutes

Cook Time: 5 minutes

Ingredients

- 4 tablespoons of almond butter

- 1oz of cream cheese

- 4 tablespoons of coconut butter

- 1 tablespoon of cocoa powder

- 2 tablespoons of sugar-free syrup

- 16g of dark chocolate

Instructions

- Add all the ingredients other than coconut butter in some microwave-safe dish.

- Microwave in intervals of 15 seconds, stirring frequently, until chocolate and the cream cheese has melted and all the ingredients have incorporated fully.

- Add coconut butter, then mix all together fully.

- Spoon the batter into 12 portions in a mini-muffin tray.

- Pop these into a freezer for about 1 hour and they will be set up. Enjoy.

Nutrients per one serving: Calories 86, Total fat 7g, Total carbs 3g, protein 2g, cholesterol 3mg, sodium 21mg

Blackberry Coconut Fat Bombs

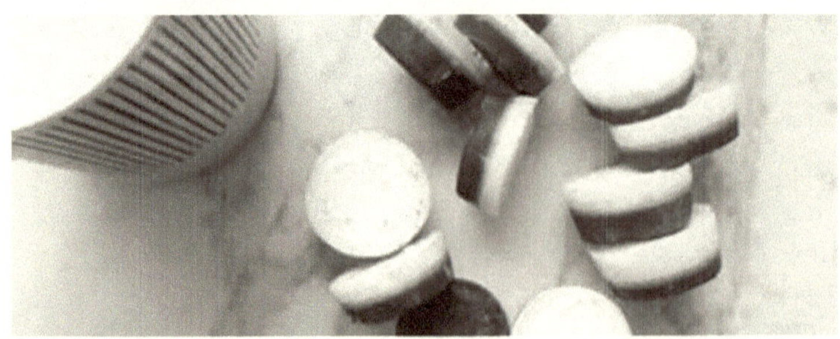

Serving: 6 people

Total Time: 10 minutes

Ingredients

*   1 cup of coconut butter

*   1/2 cup of frozen blackberries can

*   1/2 teaspoon of Sweat leaf Stevia drops

*   1/4 teaspoon of vanilla powder or a 1/2 teaspoon of vanilla extract

*   1 tablespoon of lemon juice

*   1 cup of coconut oil

Instructions

*   Place the coconut oil, coconut butter, and blackberries in a pot then heat over a medium heat until they are well combined.

*   In some food processor or a small blender, add the berry mix and the remaining ingredients. Begin to process until they are smooth.

*   Spread out into some small pan readily lined with a parchment paper

*   Refrigerate for one hour.

*   Remove from the container then cut into squares.

*   Store while covered in a refrigerator.

Nutrients per one serving: Calories 170 Calories from Fat 168, Total Fat 18.7g, Total carbohydrates 3g, Dietary Fiber 2.3g, Protein 1.1g

Chocolate Coconut Candies

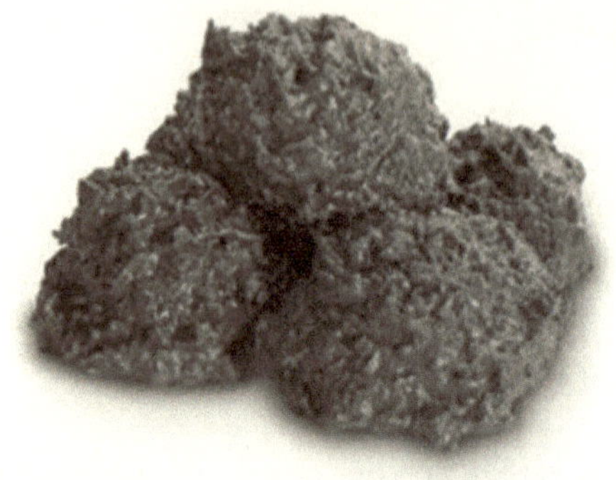

Serving: 20 mini cups

Ingredients

Coconut Candies:

- 1/2 cup of coconut butter

- 1/2 cup of Kelapo coconut oil

- 1/2 cup of shredded coconut, unsweetened

- 3 tbsps. of powdered Swerve Sweetener

Chocolate Topping:

- 1 & 1/2 ounces of Cocoa Butter

- 1 ounce of unsweetened chocolate

- 1/4 cup of powdered Swerve Sweetener

- 1/4 cup of cocoa powder

- 1/4 tsp of vanilla extract

Instructions

- For the candies, line mini-muffin pan using 20 mini paper liners.

- Combine the coconut butter and the coconut oil in some small saucepan placed over low heat. Combine well until melted then stir in the shredded coconut and the sweetener until combined.

- Divide the mixture among your prepared mini muffin cups then freeze until firm, for about 30 minutes.

- For the chocolate coating, just combine the cocoa butter and the unsweetened chocolate in a bowl placed over a pan of simmering water. Stir until melted.

- Stir in the sifted powdered sweetener, and stir in the cocoa powder, until it is smooth.

- Remove from the heat then stir in the vanilla extract.

- Spoon the chocolate topping over the chilled coconut candies then allow to set, for about 15 minutes.

Nutrients per one serving: 240 Calories, 2g Protein, 25g Fat, 5g Carbohydrate, 0mg Cholesterol, 6mg Sodium, 4g Dietary Fiber

Ginger Fat Bombs

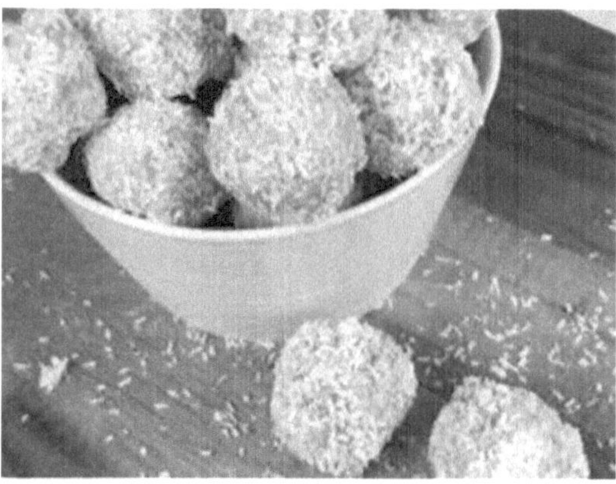

Serving: 10 people

Prep Time: 10 min

Ingredients

*   75g / 2.6oz of coconut butter

*   75g / 2.6oz of coconut oil

*   25g / 1oz of shredded/desiccated coconut

*   1 tsp of granulated sweetener

*   1/2-1 tsp of ginger powder

Instructions

*   Mix all your ingredients in some pouring jug until your sweetener becomes dissolved.

*   Pour into some silicon molds or some ice block trays then refrigerate for around 10 minutes.

Nutrients per one serving: Calories 120, Total Fat 12.8g, Fiber 1.4g, Sugars 0.1g, Protein 0.5g

Lemon Clouds

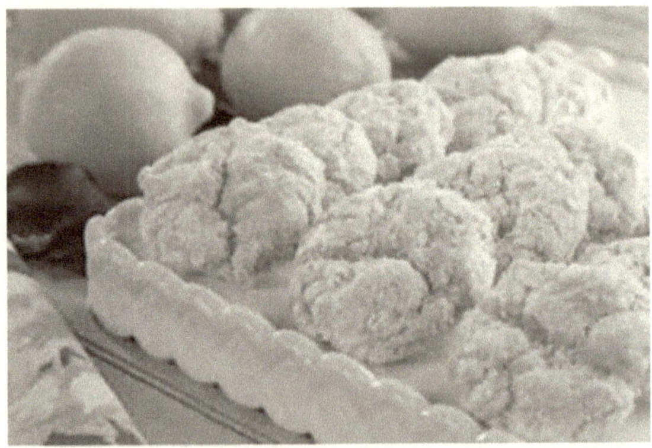

Serving: 16 bombs

Prep Time: 10 min

Ingredients

- Lemon, squeezed

- 1 tsp of lemon extract

- Sweetener to taste

- Silicone mold or ice cube tray

- 4 tbsps. of butter

- 4 tbsps. of virgin coconut oil

- 2oz of cream cheese

- 4 tbsps. of heavy cream

Instructions

- Begin with cream cheese, by heating it in short bursts. Add in the butter and the coconut oil then whisk until well blended. Add the cream last then whisk.

- Squeeze in the lemon then watch for the pesky seeds. Add extract if needed.

- Sweeten so as to taste.

- Carefully pour into the tray then balance in the freezer overnight.

- Pop them from the tray in the next morning.

Nutrients per one serving: Calories: 74.7, Fat: 8g, Protein: 0.3g, Carbs: 0.7g, Fiber: 0.8g, Sugars: 0.3g

Orange Pecan Butter Fat Bombs

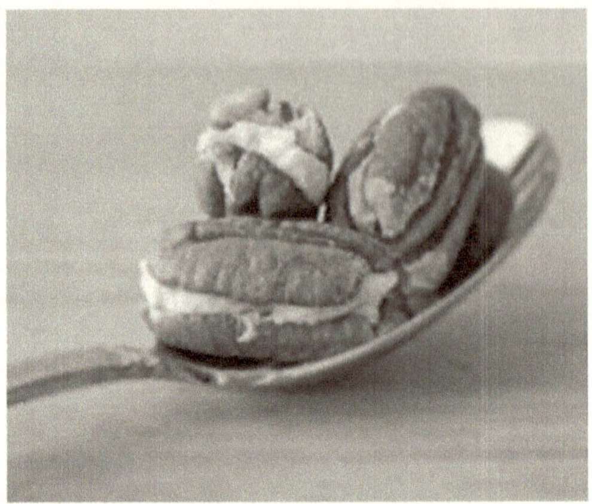

Serving: 2 people

Prep Time: 10 min

Ingredients

- 4 toasted pecan halves

- 1/2 tbsp. of unsalted grass-fed butter

- 1/2 tsp of orange zest, finely grated

- 1 pinch of sea salt

Instructions

• Toast your pecans at 350° in an oven for about 8-10 minutes, then keep aside to cool.

• Soften butter, then add orange zest then mix well until it becomes smooth and creamy.

• Spread half of the butter-orange mixture in two pecan halves. Sprinkle using sea salt then enjoy.

Nutrients per one serving: Calories 89, Net carbs 1

Raspberry Cheesecake Truffles

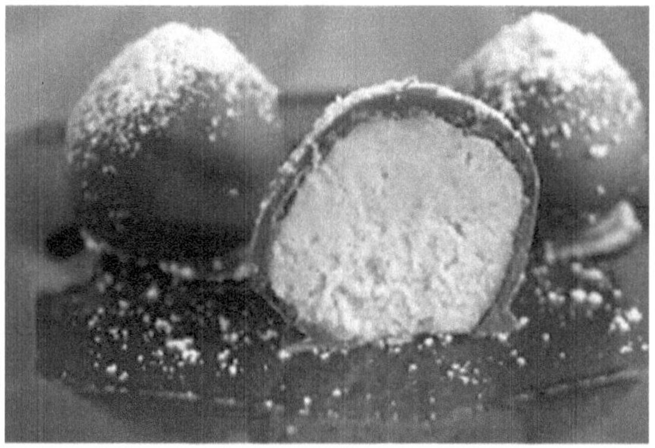

Serving: 48 balls

Prep Time: 3 hours

Ingredients

- 8 ounces of softened cream cheese

- Teaspoons of raspberry extract

- Few drops natural food coloring, red

- 1/4 cup of melted coconut oil

- 1/2 cup of powdered Swerve

- 2 tablespoons of heavy cream

- A teaspoon of vanilla stevia

- Pinch of salt

- 1 1/2 cup of chocolate chips, sugar-free

Instructions

- In your stand mixer, blend cream cheese and the Swerve until smooth.

- Add stevia, salt, cream, and raspberry extract, the natural food coloring until combined well.

- Slowly add coconut oil then proceed with blending on high till it becomes incorporated.

- Scrape down edges of your bowl so as to ensure it becomes mixed well.

- Refrigerate the mixture for about 1 hour.

- Use1 1/4 inch of mini cookie scoop, then scoop batter into a baking sheet lined with parchment paper.

- Freeze for 1 hour then coat using melted chocolate.

- Drop a cheesecake truffle into the melted chocolate then place bake on a lined pan.

- Refrigerate for extra one hour.

Nutrients per one serving: Calories : 81, Sat Fat: 5.9g, Fat: 8.6g, Cholesterol: 20mg, Carbs: 1g, Fiber: 0g, Sodium: 63mg, Protein: 1g, Sugars: .5g

Cheesy Pesto Fat Bombs

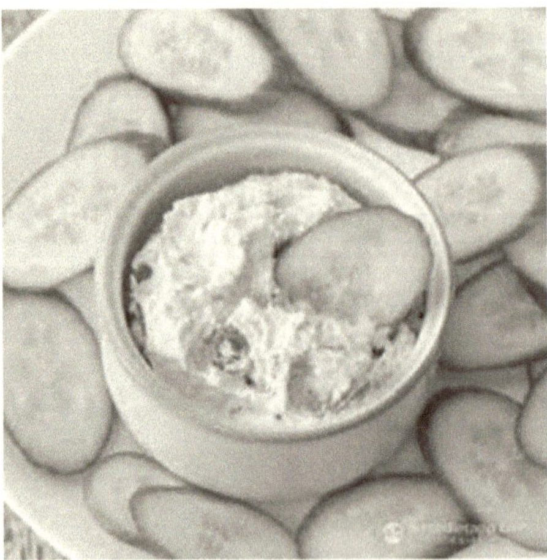

Serving: 8 people

Prep Time: 5 min

Ingredients

- 10 sliced olives

- Salt, pepper to taste (optional)

- 1 cup of full-fat cream cheese

- 2 tbsps. of basil pesto

- ½ cup of grated Parmesan cheese

Instructions

- Place all your ingredients in some bowl, cream cheese, pesto, parmesan, and olives. Mix by use of a spatula until they are well combined.

- Slice your cucumber or the other fresh vegetables which you are planning to serve it with.

- Place remaining dip in some airtight container put in a fridge for a week.

Nutrients per one serving: Total Carbs 1.6g, Fiber 0.3g, Protein 4.3g, Fat 12.9g, Magnesium 37mg, Potassium 50mg

Cream Cheese and Peanut Butter Fat Bomb

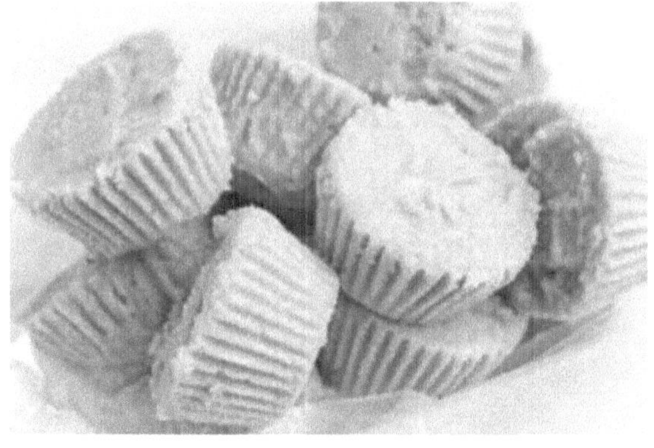

Serving: 14 pieces

Prep Time: 10 min

Ingredients

- 2 Tablespoons of sour cream

- 4 Tablespoons of softened cream cheese

- 1 cup of heavy whipping cream

- 3 Tablespoons of BP2 peanut butter, powdered

- 2 Tablespoons of Splenda

Instructions

- Whip heavy whipping cream for it to be light and airy. Add the remaining ingredients and mix well.

- Spoon into some silicone candy mold tray to make 14 portions then freeze overnight.

- Serve them partially frozen or allow to defrost completely for a fluffy treat.

Nutrients per one serving: Calories 82, Total fat 8g, Cholesterol 24mg, Sodium 29mg, Totals carbs 1g, Protein 1g

Walnut Chocolate and Orange Fat Bombs

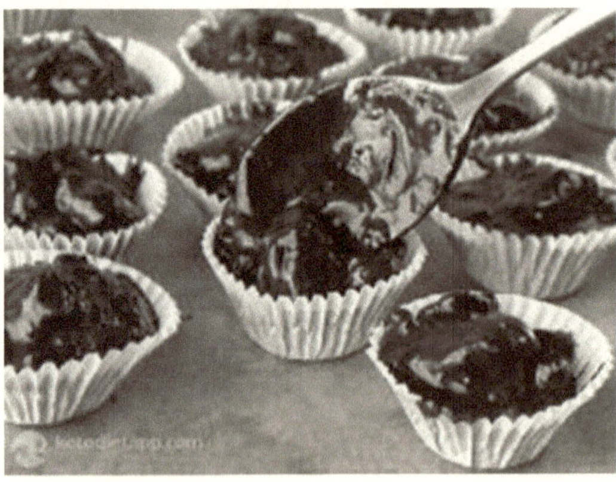

Serving: 25 pieces

Prep Time: 15 min

Cook Time: 1Hr

Ingredients

- 125g of dark chocolate

- 1 tsp of cinnamon

- 10-15 drops stevia

- ¼ cup of extra virgin coconut oil.9 oz.)

- 1⅓ cup of chopped walnuts

- ½ - 1 tbsp. of orange peel

Instructions

- Melt chocolate in some water bath then adds coconut oil and the cinnamon. Sweeten using stevia if it is needed then mix well.

- Add the fresh orange peel and the orange food extract.

- Add your roughly chopped walnuts then mix in well.

- Spoon your mixture into some small paper muffin or some candy cups.

- Place in a fridge for some couple of hours or till solid. Keep at room temperature.

Nutrients per one serving: Total carbs 2.4g, Fiber 0.93g, Protein 1.5g, Fat 8.4g, Potassium 64mg

Spiced Refrigerator Candy

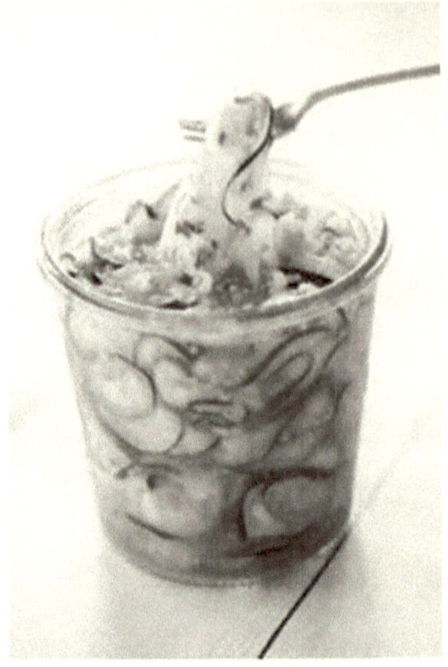

Serving: 6 people

Prep Time: 10 min

Cook Time: 5 min

Ingredients

- 8 ounces of cream cheese

- 1/2 tsp (1g) of cloves, ground

- 1/2 tsp (1g) of nutmeg, freshly ground

- 3/4 cup of coconut oil

- 1/2 cup of 'Swerve'

- 2g of fresh ginger, grated

- 2g of cinnamon, ground

Instructions

- Add all the ingredients to food processor, except liquid coconut oil.

- Turn on your food processor.

- As the processor runs, pour coconut oil into cream cheese slowly.

- Divide this into 6 smaller cups.

- Refrigerate.

Nutrients per one serving: Calories 372, fat 36.98g, Protein 2.32g, Carbs 18.65g, Fiber 0.28g

Chocolate Mousse

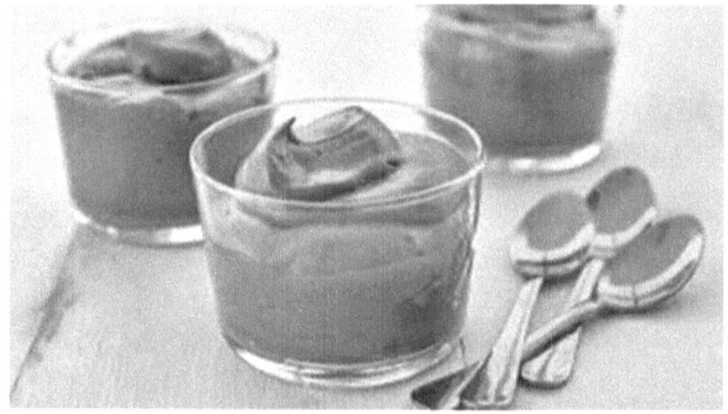

Serving: 4 people

Prep Time: 5 min

Ingredients

- ½ tsp of cinnamon

- 6-12 drops of liquid stevia extract

- Shredded coconut for garnish

- 1 cup of creamed coconut milk

- 3 tbsps. of raw cocoa powder

Instructions

•	Put a coconut milk can into your fridge overnight. Once thick, put it into a bowl.

•	Whip in raw cocoa powder.

•	Add in cinnamon and stevia.

•	Whip until it's smooth and creamy.

•	Place in serving glass then garnish using some pinch of shredded coconut. Enjoy!

Nutrients per one serving: Total Carbs 13.5g, Fiber 5.8g, Protein 6.2g, Fat 42.9g, Magnesium 75mg, Potassium 520mg

Chocolate Fat Bombs

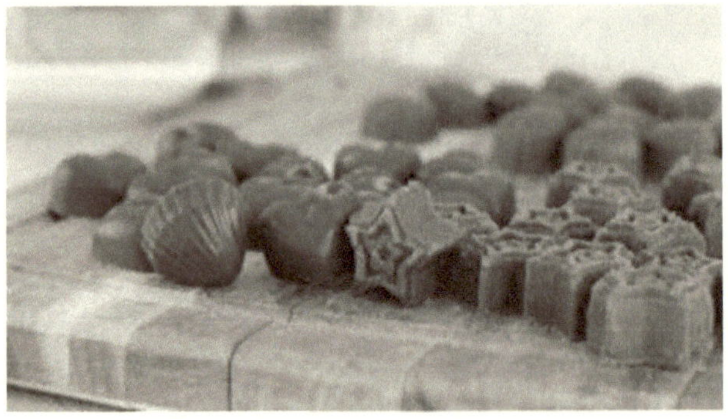

Serving: 14 people

Prep Time: 10 min

Ingredients

•	125g / 4.5oz of coconut oil

•	25g / 1oz of unsweetened cocoa powder

•	1 tbsp. of granulated sweetener

•	1-2 tbsps. Of tahini paste

*   25g / 1oz of walnut halves

Instructions

*   Warm your coconut oil until becomes melted.

*   Add the other ingredients (other than walnuts) then allow to cool so that ingredients do not settle and sink to the bottom of your fat bomb.

*   Pour into the ice cube trays then refrigerate until it is semi-set.

*   Once it's almost set, put half walnut on the top of every fat bomb.

Nutrients per one serving: Calories 119, Total fat 12.6g, Total Carbs 1.2g, Protein 1.4g

Bulletproof Fat Bombs

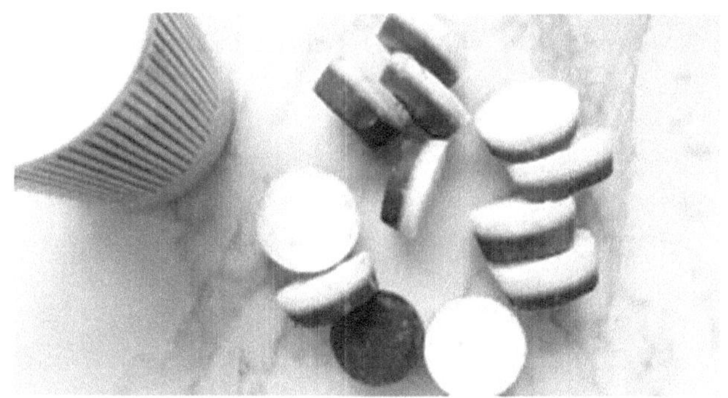

Prep Time: 15 min

Cook Time: 1 hr. 30 min

Ingredients

*   1 cup of creamed coconut milk

*   10-15 drops of liquid stevia extract

*   ½ cup of strong brewed coffee

*   ¼ cup of grass-fed butter

*   2 tbsps. of MCT oil

- 2 tbsps. of raw cocoa powder

- ¼ cup of Swerve or Erythritol

- 1tsp of rum extract

Instructions

- Put softened creamed coconut milk, butter, MCT oil, and the cocoa powder.

- Add the powdered Erythritol and the stevia into a blender then pulse until smooth.

- Pour in a prepared coffee then pulse again until it becomes smooth. Pour into ice-cream maker then process while following manufacturer's instructions.

- Spoon 2 tablespoons of ice-cream into the ice tray which is good for making of fat bomb shapes.

- Place in a freezer for about 2-3 hours or until it becomes firm.

Nutrients per one serving: Total carbs 0.7g, fiber 0.2g, protein 0.8g, fat 8.1g

Peanut Butter Fudge

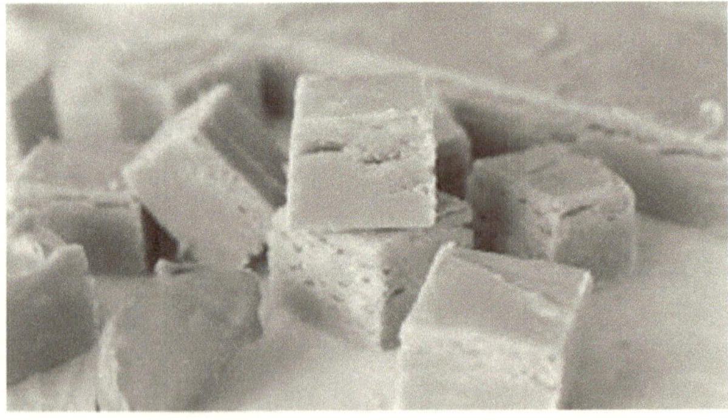

Serving: 12 people

Prep Time: 5 min

Ingredients

- 1 cup of unsweetened peanut butter

- 1/4 cup of unsweetened cocoa powder

- 1 cup of coconut oil

- 1/4 cup of vanilla almond milk, unsweetened

- Pinch salt (optional)

- 2 teaspoons of vanilla liquid stevia (optional)

- 2 tablespoons of coconut oil, melted

- 2 tablespoons of Swerve

Instructions

- Slightly melt/soften the peanut butter and the coconut oil in some microwave or a low heat on a stove.

- Add it to a blender and the remaining ingredients.

- Blend until well combined.

- Pour into your loaf pan with parchment paper lining.

- Refrigerate for 2 hours until set.

- If you are using chocolate sauce, just whisk the ingredients together then drizzle over the fudge after it has been set.

Nutrients per one serving: Calories 287, Fat 29.7g, Carbs 4g, Sugar 0.7g, Sodium 4mg, Fiber 1.4g, Protein 5.4g

Buttered Bacon Fat Bomb

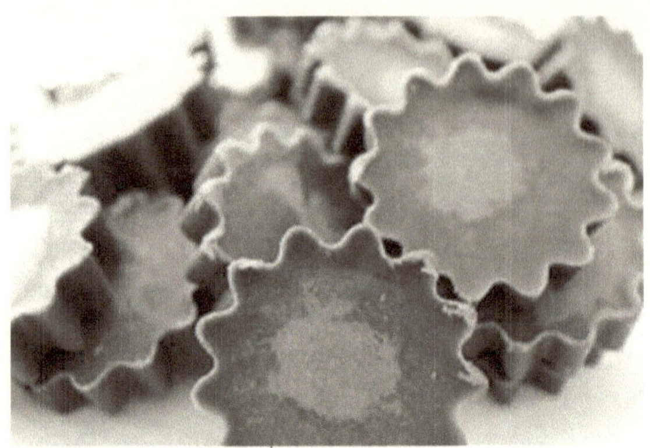

Serving: 3 fat bombs

Prep Time: 2 min

Ingredients

- 1 bacon slice

- 2 toasted & chopped pecan halves

- 1/16 serving of Keto Craisin

- 1 tablespoon of unsalted Kerrygold butter

- 1 pinch of granulated garlic (optional)

Instructions

- Divide your bacon into 3 parts. Slather each of these using 1 teaspoon of the Kerrygold unsalted butter.

- Press the butter side into your pecan pieces.

- Top each using Keto Craisin.

Nutrients per one serving: 158 Calories, 2g Protein, 17g Fat, 1g Carbohydrate, 1g Effective Carbs, trace Dietary Fiber

Indian Keto Coconut Bars

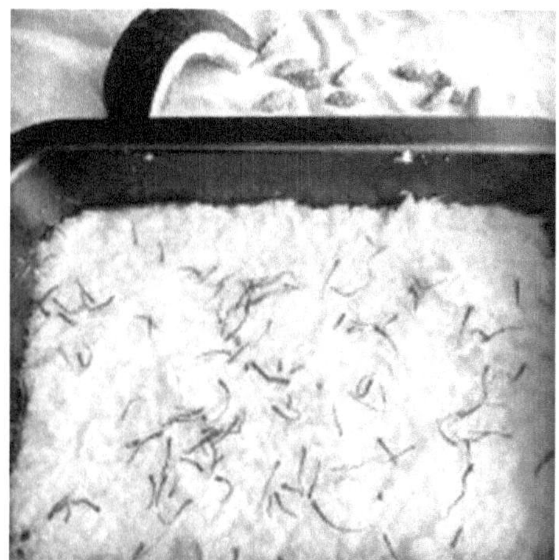

Prep Time: 35 min

Cook Time: 1hr 30 min

Ingredients

- 4 tbsps. of Erythritol

- 1 tsp of cardamom powder

- 10-20 saffron threads

- 1 ¾ cups of shredded unsweetened coconut

- 1⅓ cup of unsweetened coconut milk

- 100 ghee

Instructions

- Take some bowl then mix shredded coconut with the 300 ml of coconut milk in it. Keep the mixture aside for about 30 minutes.

- Add the remaining 20 ml of coconut milk then add saffron threads and erythritol. Mix these properly for sugar to dissolve.

- Heat a wok then melt your ghee in it. Add coconut mixture, then keep mixing and ensuring flame is maintained at low and your mixture doesn't stick to the surface. Continue mixing for about 5-7 minutes.

•   Add Elaichi / cardamom powder then cook your mixture for an extra 5 minutes.

•   Take some baking tray/ barfi tray, butter it then spread your mixture evenly, until a thickness of 1 cm is formed. Freeze this for about 2 to 2½ hours.

•   Cut the small squares according to own liking, and you will have your barfi ready. Refrigerate this for 5 days.

Nutrients per one serving: Total Carbs 2.9g, Fiber 1.5g, Protein 2.2g, Fat 12.1g, Magnesium 15mg, Potassium 82mg

Mocha Vanilla Fat Bomb Pops

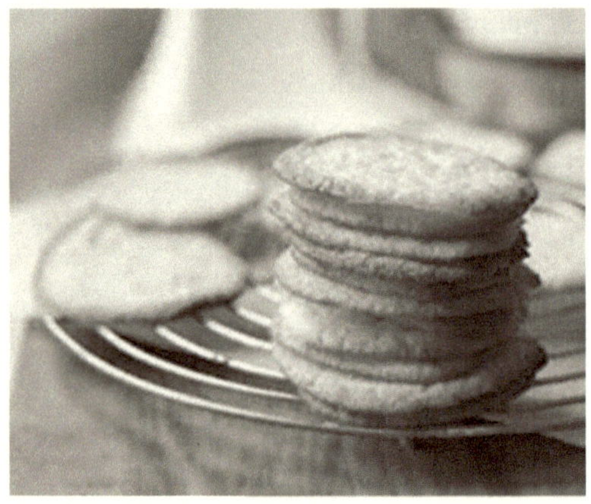

Serving: 6 people

Prep Time: 10 min

Ingredients

•   2 tbsps. of heavy cream

•   1/2 tsp of vanilla extract

•   4 tbsps. of coconut oil

- 1/2 tbsp. of unsweetened cocoa powder

- 4 tbsps. of unsalted butter

- 1/2 tsp of coffee extract

- Stevia, to taste

Instructions

- Make vanilla layer:

- Soften butter in a microwave until liquefied.

- Add the heavy cream then stir. Keep aside.

- Once cooled, add in vanilla then blend well.

- Pour vanilla mixture into the muffin liners/tins. Place into your refrigerator until it is firm.

 Make mocha layer:

- Mix coconut oil, coffee extract, cocoa powder and stevia.

- Remove the vanilla layer from the fridge then pour in mocha mixture, while filling the cups to the top.

- Add the popsicle sticks then freeze for 20 to 30 minutes.

Nutrition information per serving: 167 Calories; trace Protein, 19g Fat,.5g Dietary Fiber, 1g Carbohydrate

Low-carb pumpkin keto pastille

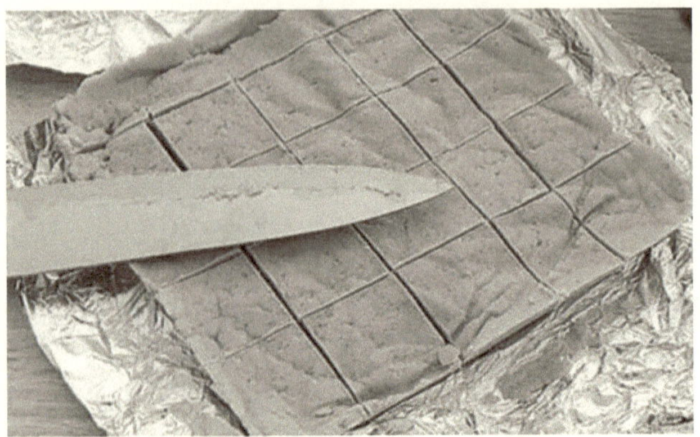

Servings 20

Total Time: 10 minutes + 2 hours for freezing

Ingredients:

- 1 ½ cup coconut oil

- 1 cup pumpkin puree

- ¼ tsp ground nutmeg

- 1 tsp cinnamon

Cooking process:

1.   Cover the baking sheet with aluminum foil.

2.   Pour coconut oil into a saucepan, heat until completely dissolved. Cool it down.

3.   Add the pumpkin puree and spices, and stir it.

4.   Put the mass in a mold and evenly distribute it throughout the volume. Cover it with parchment and to press down with hands.

5.   Remove parchment and leave pastille in the refrigerator for 2 hours.

6.   Remove from the mold and cut into 20 squares.

Nutrients per one serving:

Calories: 109.1 | Fats: 10.6 g. | Carbohydrates: 2.1 g. | Proteins: 1.21 g.

Coconut and almond fat bombs

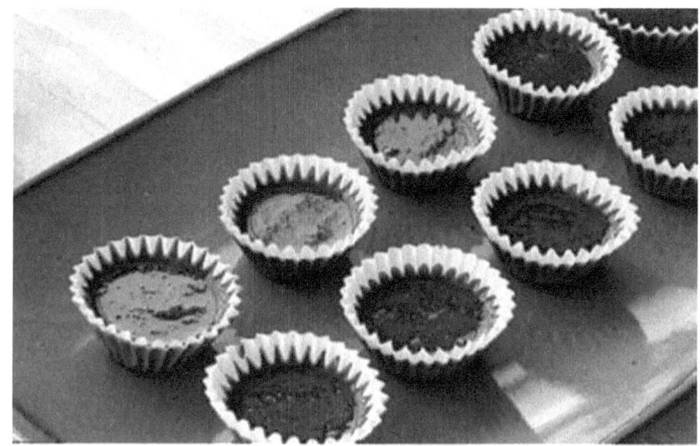

Servings 8-10

Total Time: 10 minutes + 20 minutes for cooling

Ingredients:

- ½ cup almond oil

- ½ cup coconut oil

- 3 tbsp cocoa powder

- ½ cup erythritol

Cooking process:

1.   In a fire-resistant container, mix coconut oil and almond oil. Warm up in the microwave for 50 seconds. Mix to uniformity.

2.   Add cocoa and erythritol, and mix it all.

3.   Pour the mass into paper or silicone molds for cupcakes, cool while 20 minutes in the refrigerator.

Fat Bombs of coconut oil

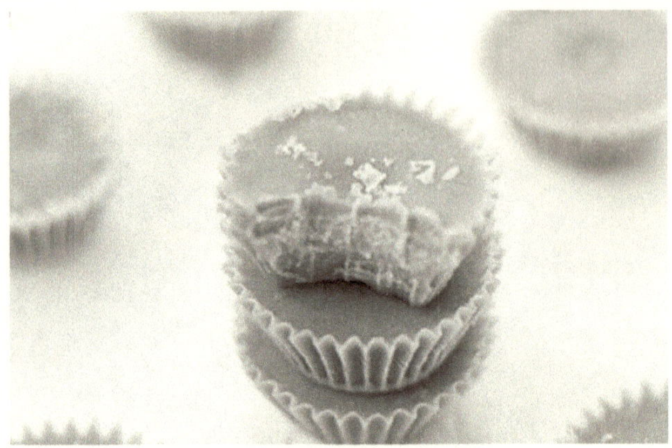

Servings 10

Total Time: 10 minutes + 2 hours for freezing

Ingredients:

- ½ cup coconut oil

- ½ cup cream

- 120 g cream cheese

- 1 tsp color vanilla

- 12 drops liquid stevia

Cooking process:

1. Put all the ingredients in the blender, and mix for 1 minute until uniformity.

2. Pour the mass into the silicone molds and leave it in the freezer for 2 hours.

3. Remove fat bombs from molds and store them in a plastic container in

the refrigerator.

Nutrients per one serving:

Calories: 178 | Fats: 18.9 g. | Carbohydrates: 0.94 g. | Proteins: 1.05 g.

Keto truffles with pistachios

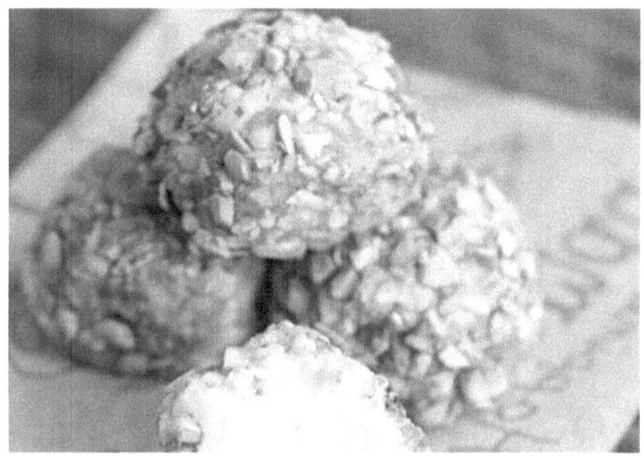

Servings 10

Total Time: 10 minutes + 20 minutes for frozen

Ingredients:

- 1 cup soft mascarpone

- ¼ tsp vanilla

- 3 tbsp stevia

- ¼ cup chopped pistachios

Cooking process:

1.   In a bowl, mix the mascarpone, vanilla, and sweetener until uniformity.

2.   Divide the mass into equal portions and form balls with a diameter of 5-7 cm.

3.   Put out pistachios on a dish. Roll the truffles in the pistachios and

leave in the freezer for 20 minutes.

Nutrients per one serving:

Calories: 250 | Fats: 21 g. | Carbohydrates: 4.6 g. | Proteins: 9.8 g.

Coconut fat bombs with a lemon peel

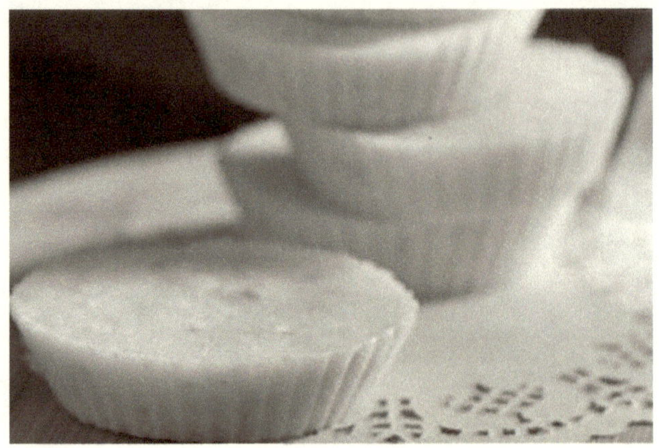

Servings 6

Total Time: 10 minutes + 20 minutes for cooling

Ingredients:

*   100 g coconut oil

*   60 g coconut flakes

*   1 tsp stevia

*   2 tbsp lemon peel

Cooking process:

*   Mix coconut oil until uniformity. In a bowl, mix all ingredients to receive a dense mass.

*   Form round bombs of 20 g each, and lay out in a container.

- Leave in the refrigerator for 20 minutes for cooling.

Nutrients per one serving:

Calories: 126 | Fats: 14.2 g. | Carbohydrates: 0.31 g. | Proteins: 0.07 g.

Coconut Keto Bombs

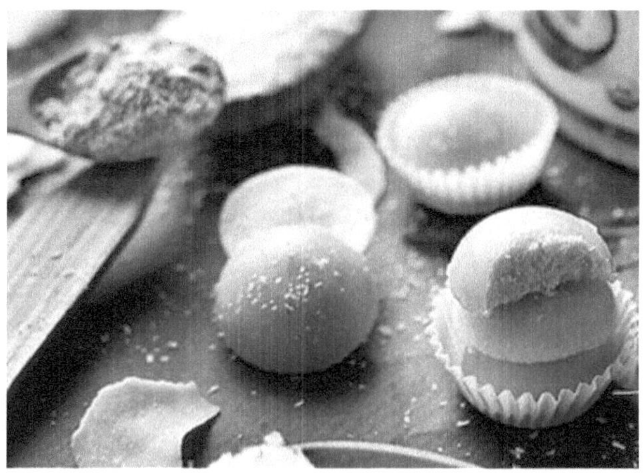

Servings 12

Total Time: 10 minutes + 1 hour for freezing

Ingredients:

- 100 g coconut oil

- 100 g coconut chips

- 100 g coconut manna

- 15 g peanut powder

Cooking process:

- Mix all ingredients in a deep bowl and pre-heat in a water bath until uniformity.

- Pour the creamy mass into silicone molds for cupcakes. Leave in the refrigerator for 1 hour to freeze.

Nutrients per one serving:

Calories: 37.7 | Fats: 3.7 g. | Carbohydrates: 0.6 g. | Proteins: 0.28 g.

Keto chocolate sausage

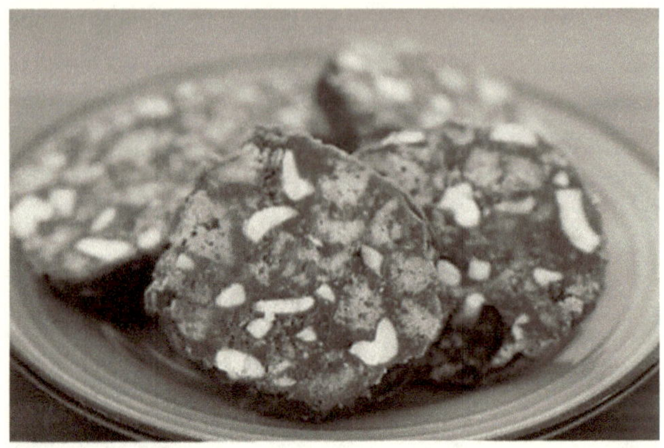

Servings 8-10

Total Time: 25 minutes + 4 hours for cooling

Ingredients:

- 200 g coconut oil

- 85 g keto bread

- 2 tbsp stevia

- 3 tbsp cocoa powder

- 1 tsp vanilla

- 50 g nuts

- Parchment for baking

Cooking process:

1. Cut the bread into slices and dry it in a dry frying pan. Chop the nuts.

2.   Melt the butter in the microwave for 1 minute. Add the vanilla.

3.   Mix cocoa and stevia, add crushed bread, butter, and nuts. Mix well. Leave in the refrigerator for 25 minutes.

4.   Put a cooled mass on a parchment and form a long sausage, roll up it and leave in the refrigerator for 4 hours. Slice into portions.

Nutrients per one serving:

Calories: 114 | Fats: 11.5 g. | Carbohydrates: 2.36 g. | Proteins: 1.35 g.

Peanut balls in coconut flakes

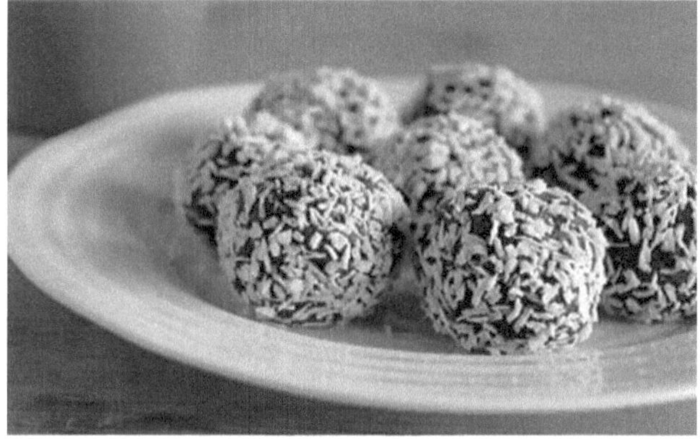

Servings 12

Total Time: 5 minutes + 10 hours for freezing

Ingredients:

*   3 tbsp peanut butter

*   3 tsp cocoa powder

*   2 tsp erythritol powder

*   2 tsp almond flour

*   ½ cup coconut flakes

Cooking process:

1.   In a bowl, mix the peanut butter, erythritol, cocoa, and flour. Cool the received mass in the freezer for 1 hour.

2.   Divide mix into equal portions by a teaspoon. Form the balls and roll them in coconut flakes.

3.   Leave keto bombs for 10 hours in the refrigerator.

Nutrients per one serving:

Calories: 35.1 | Fats: 3.1 g. | Carbohydrates: 0.9 g. | Proteins: 0.97 g.

Neapolitan fat bombs

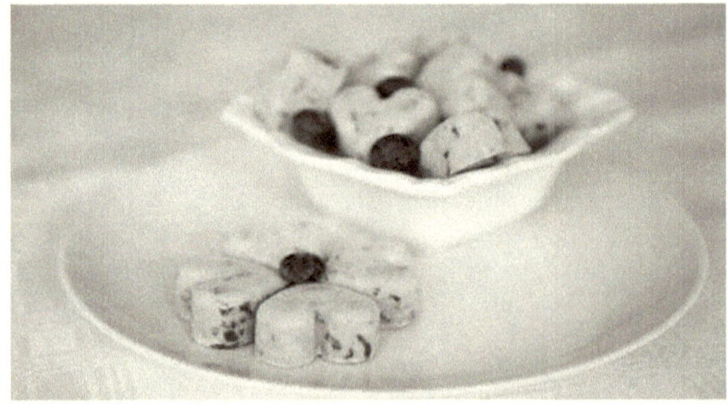

Servings 6-8

Total Time: 10 minutes + 2 hours for freezing

Ingredients:

- ½ cup coconut oil

- ½ cup sour cream

- ½ cup cream cheese

- 200 g butter

- 22 drops liquid stevia

- 3 tbsp cocoa powder

- 2 tbsp erythritol

- 1 tsp vanilla

- 2 strawberries

Cooking process:

1.   Put all the ingredients in the blender (except cocoa, vanilla, and strawberries). Mix them for 1 minute.

2.   Divide the mass into 3 cups. Add cocoa in the first cup, add vanilla in the second cup, and add crushed strawberry in the third cup.

3.   Into a silicone mold, pour the chocolate mass and leave in the freezer for 25 minutes.

4.   Pour the vanilla over the chocolate layer and freeze it. Pour the strawberry layer on the top and leave in the freezer for 1 hour.

5.   Lay out on a dish when serving.

Nutrients per one serving:

Calories: 103 | Fats: 10.9 g. | Carbohydrates: 0.61 g. | Proteins: 0.52 g.

Low-carb lemon soufflé

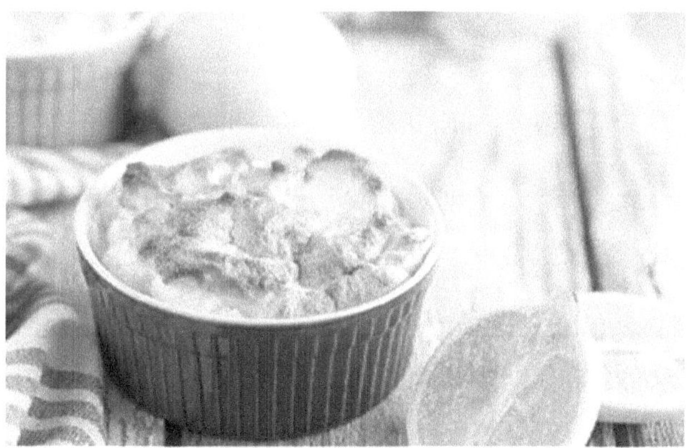

Servings 4

Total Time: 30 minutes

Ingredients:

- 250 g ricotta cheese

- 2 eggs

- ¼ cup erythritol

- 2 tsp lemon peel

- 1 tbsp lemon juice

- 1 tsp seeds of poppies

- 1 ½ tsp vanilla

Cooking process:

1. Heat the oven to 200 °C. To separate yolks from proteins. Beat proteins by the mixer to dense peaks, add 3 tablespoons of erythritol and mix them for 1 minute again.

2. Add the ricotta cheese and the remaining erythritol to the egg yolks. Mix until uniformity.

3. Add lemon peel, juice, vanilla and poppy seeds to the cheese mass. Mix very well.

4. Connect all ingredients of the two bowls and mix well.

5. Grease ramekins and lay out the mass for the soufflé, level the top with a spoon. Bake in the oven for 20 minutes.

Nutrients per one serving:

Calories: 156 | Fats: 11.01 g. | Carbohydrates: 2.6 g. | Proteins: 10.3 g.

Coconut bombs with rice balls

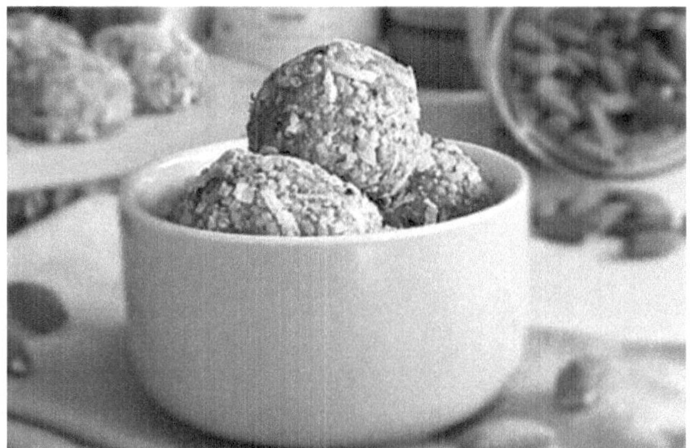

Servings 15

Total Time: 20 minutes + 15 minutes for freezing

Ingredients:

* 2 cups coconut flakes

* ⅓ cup coconut oil

* 2 tbsp honey

* 1 tsp vanilla

* 3 tbsp rice balls

Cooking process:

1.   Put the coconut flakes, coconut oil, honey and vanilla in the blender. Mix them at high speed for 1 minute to uniformity.

2.   Cover a tray with parchment. Divide the mass into equal parts by a tablespoon and make the small balls.

3.   Roll ready bombs in rice balls and put in a freezer for 15 minutes for freezing. Store them in a refrigerator in a sealed container.

Chocolates with nuts without sugar

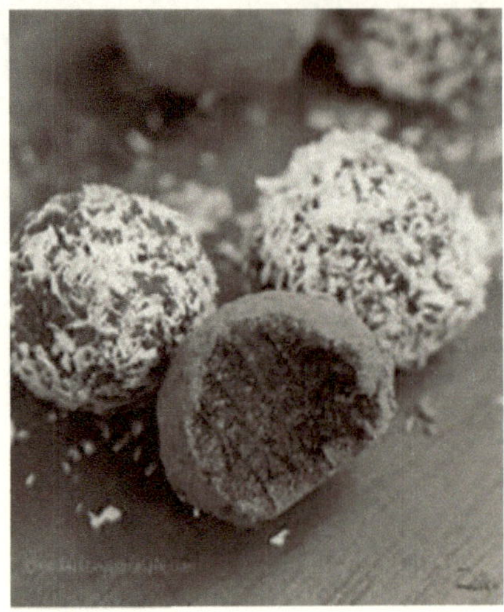

Servings 8-10

Total Time: 10 minutes + 4 hours for cooling

Ingredients:

- 100 g butter

- 5 tbsp coconut flakes

- 25 g nuts

- 1 tbsp cocoa powder

- 1 tsp vanilla

- 1 tsp erythritol

Cooking process:

1.   Put the butter in a saucepan and melt over low fire. Add coconut flakes, cocoa, vanilla, erythritol and crushed nuts. Mix it all.

2. Put the mass in a silicone mold and level it with a spoon.

3. Leave in the refrigerator for 3-4 hours for cooling.

4. Cut into small squares when serving.

Nutrients per one serving:

Calories: 53 | Fats: 5.8 g. | Carbohydrates: 0.88 g. | Proteins: 0.35 g.

Keto bombs with coconut cream

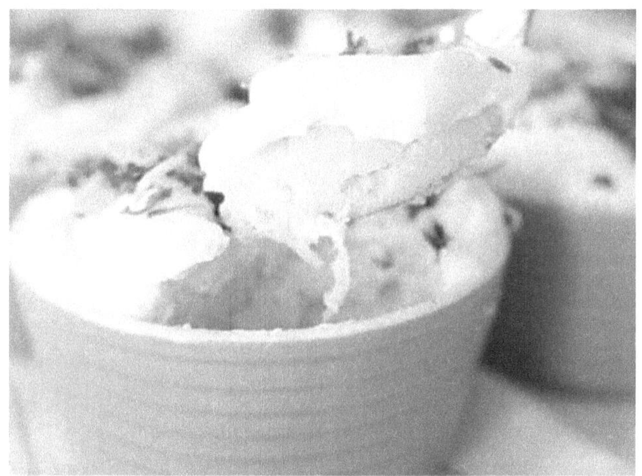

Servings 4-6

Total Time: 20 minutes + 1 hour for freezing

Ingredients for the base:

*   5 tbsp butter

*   ¼ cup stevia

*   ½ cup almond flour

*   ¼ cup coconut flakes

Ingredients for cream:

- 1 cup fat cream

- 2 egg yolks

- ¼ cups coconut flour

- ½ cups water

- ¼ cup stevia

- 1 tsp vanilla

Ingredients for decor:

- 2 tbsp coconut flakes

- 1 tsp vanilla

Cooking process:

1.   Put the butter in a saucepan and melt over low fire. Add the stevia, and mix it all.

2.   Add almond flour and flakes to the creamy mass. Stir well until uniformity.

3.   Pour the dough into the cupcake molds, level it and cool down.

4.   Separate yolks from proteins. Mix yolks with coconut flour, add water to get a thick mass. In another bowl, whisk the proteins until dense peaks.

5.   Put the cream in a saucepan and heat it over low fire. Add vanilla, whipped yolks and proteins, stir until uniformity. To cool cream and lay out it on the base. Leave in the refrigerator for 60 minutes.

6.   Mix coconut flakes with vanilla and fry in a dry frying pan. Decorate the bombs with fried flakes.

Nutrients per one serving:

Calories: 583 | Fats: 57.6 g. | Carbohydrates: 7.2 g. | Proteins: 9.2 g..

Chapter 3: KETO BREAD

What is Keto Bread?

We are often afraid of bread because they are often high in starch, high in fat and provide plenty of calories. This is extremely harmful to people who are overweight, obese, type 2 diabetes and many other chronic diseases. However, keto bread is different! This is healthy food suitable for people who are practicing ketogenic diets, paleo, and people who are sensitive to gluten.

Keto bread is a mixture of almond flour or coconut powder, eggs, healthy fats, and xanthan gum. It has the same ingredients as regular wheat bread in texture but has about 20 times fewer carbs than regular bread.

If you are following a ketogenic diet, you should know the keto recipes below! At the same time, this is a very healthy bread recipe for people on the paleo diet and gluten-free people.

Let us now look at some tasty ketogenic recipes:

Kale Crackers

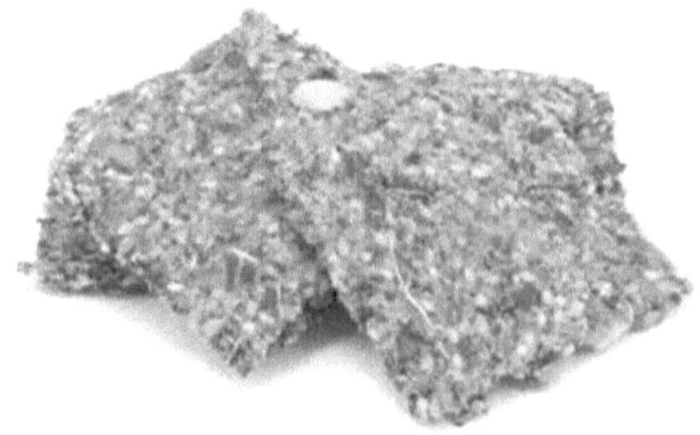

Serves: 20

Ingredients:

- 2 cup Almonds, soaked overnight, drained and rinsed, finely chopped

- 1 cup Coconut Flour

- 3/4 cup Nutritional Yeast

- 1 tsp Chipotle

- 1 tsp Smoked Paprika

- 1 cup Ground Flax Seeds, soaked in 1 cup water

- 1 bunch Kale, chopped

- Himalayan Salt, to taste

- Black Pepper, to taste

Directions:

- Line a baking sheet with parchment paper and set aside.

- Combine the almonds, coconut flour, nutritional yeast, chipotle, and paprika. Add the kale and mix well.

- Pour in the flax and water mixture, season with salt and pepper, and knead the dough.

- Transfer the dough to a sheet of parchment paper, cover with another sheet and roll out the dough. Cut into crackers, place them on the prepared sheet and dehydrate at 290F / 145C for half an hour. Reduce the heat to 245F / 118C and dehydrate the crackers for about 8 hours, flipping halfway through.

Nutrients per one serving:

Calories: 88, Total Fat: 10.2 g, Saturated Fat: 1.5 g, Carbs: 5.4 g, Sugars: 0.4 g, Protein: 4.6 g

Chili Crackers

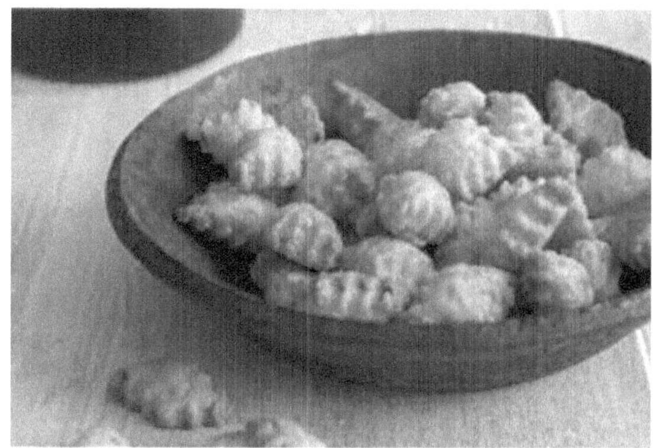

Serves: 30 crackers

Ingredients:

- ¾ cup Almond Flour

- ¼ cup Coconut Flour

- ¼ cup Flax Seed

- ½ tsp Paprika

- ½ tsp Cumin

- 1 1/2 tsp Chili Pepper Spice

- 1 tsp Onion Powder

- ½ tsp Salt

- 1 Egg

- ¼ cup Unsalted Butter

Directions:

- Preheat your oven to 350F / 175C. Line a baking sheet with parchment paper and set aside.

- Add the ingredients to your food processor and pulse until dough forms.

•   Divide the dough into two equal parts. Place one ball on a sheet of parchment pepper, cover with another sheet and roll it out. Cut into crackers and repeat the same with the other ball of dough. Transfer the crackers to the prepared baking tray.

•   Bake for about 8-10 minutes. When done, remove from the oven, leave to cool and serve.

Nutrients per one serving:

Calories: 49, Total Fat: 4.1 g, Saturated Fat: 1.2 g, Carbs: 2.8 g, Sugars: 0.1 g, Protein: 1.6 g

Almond & Flax Crackers

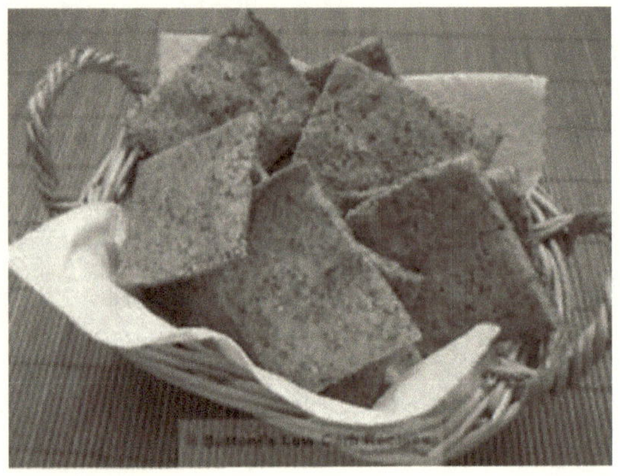

Serves: 20-24 crackers

Ingredients:

•   ½ cup Ground Flax Seeds

•   ½ cup Almond Flour

•   1 Tbsp Coconut Flour

•   2 Tbsp Shelled Hemp Seeds

•   ¼ tsp Fine Sea Salt, plus more to sprinkle on top

*   1 Egg White

*   2 Tbsp Unsalted Butter, melted

Directions:

*   Preheat your oven to 300F / 150C. Line a baking sheet with parchment paper and set aside.

*   Combine the flax, almond, and coconut flour, hemp seed, and salt. Add the egg and melted butter and mix until well combined.

*   Transfer the dough onto a sheet of parchment paper, cover with another sheet of paper and roll out the dough. Cut into crackers and arrange them on the prepared baking sheet.

*   Bake for half an hour, allow to cool and serve.

Nutrients per one serving:

Calories: 47.7, Total Fat: 5.2 g, Saturated Fat: 1 g, Carbs: 1.2 g, Sugars: 0.1 g, Protein: 1.9 g

Roasted Herb Crackers

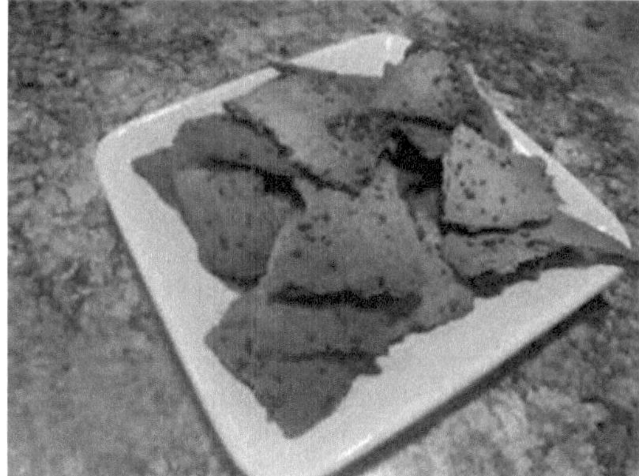

Serves: 75 crackers

Ingredients:

* ¼ cup Avocado Oil

* 10 Celery Stalks

* 1 sprig Fresh Rosemary, stem discarded

* 2 sprigs Fresh Thyme, stems discarded

* 2 Tbsp Apple Cider Vinegar

* 1 tsp Himalayan Salt

* 3 cups Ground Flax Seed

Directions:

* Preheat your oven to 225F / 110C. Line a baking sheet with parchment paper and set aside.

* Add the oil, celery, herbs, vinegar, and salt to your food processor and pulse until pureed. Add the flax and pulse again to incorporate and let sit for about 2-3 minutes until the mixture firms up.

* Transfer the batter to the prepared baking sheet, spread evenly and cut into crackers.

* Bake in the preheated oven for about an hour. Remove the parchment paper, flip the crackers and bake for one more hour. If the crackers are thick, they will need more time to bake.

* Once done, remove from the oven and leave t cool before serving.

Nutrients per one serving:

Calories: 34, Total Fat: 5.1 g, Saturated Fat: 0.3 g, Carbs: 1.5 g, Sugars: 0.3 g, Protein: 1.3 g

Garlic Breadsticks

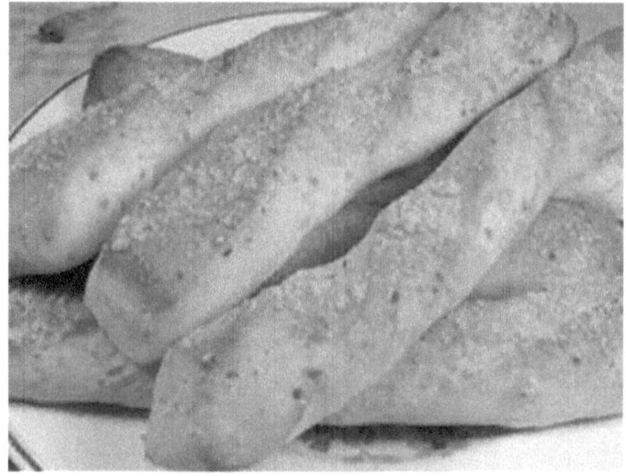

Serves: 8 breadsticks

Ingredients for the garlic butter:

- 1/4 cup Butter, softened

- 1 tsp Garlic Powder

Ingredients:

- 2 cup Almond Flour

- 1/2 Tbsp Baking Powder

- 1 Tbsp Psyllium Husk Powder

- 1/4 tsp Salt

- 3 Tbsp Butter, melted

- 1 Egg

- 1/4 cup Boiling Water

Directions:

- Preheat your oven to 400F / 200C. Line your baking sheet with parchment paper and set aside.

- Beat the butter with the garlic powder and set aside to use it for brushing.

- Combine the almond flour, baking powder, psyllium husk powder, and salt. Add the butter along with the egg and mix until well combined.

- Pour in the boiling water and mix until dough forms.

- Divide the dough into 8 equal pieces and roll them into breadsticks.

- Place on the baking sheet and bake for 15 minutes. Brush the breadsticks with the garlic butter and bake for 5 more minutes.

- Serve warm or allow to cool.

Nutrients per one serving:

Calories: 259.2, Total Fat: 24.7 g, Saturated Fat: 7.5 g, Carbs: 6.3 g, Sugars: 1.1 g, Protein: 7 g

Savory Italian Crackers

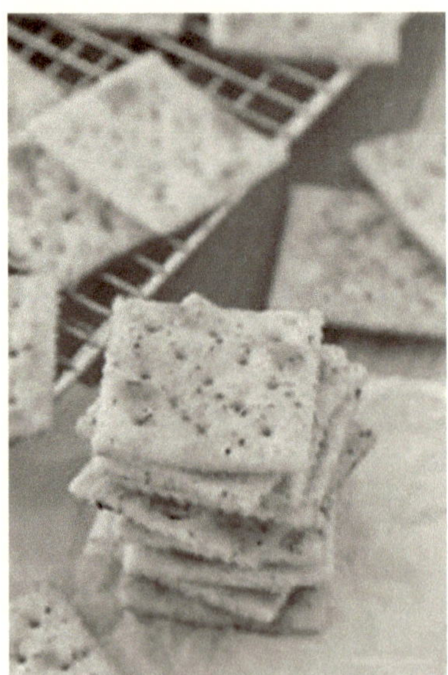

Serves: 20-30 crackers

Ingredients:

*   1 1/2 cup Almond Flour

*   1/4 tsp Garlic Powder

*   1/2 tsp Onion Powder

*   1/2 tsp Thyme

*   1/4 tsp Basil

*   1/4 tsp Oregano

*   3/4 tsp Salt

*   1 Egg

*   2 Tbsp Olive Oil

Directions:

*   Preheat your oven to 350F / 175C. Line a baking tray with parchment paper and set aside.

*   Combine all the ingredients into a food processor until dough forms.

*   Form the dough into a log and slice into thin crackers. Arrange the crackers onto the prepared baking sheet and bake for about 10-15 minutes.

*   When done, allow to cool and serve.

Nutrients per one serving:

Calories: 63.5, Total Fat: 5.8 g, Saturated Fat: 0.6 g, Carbs: 1.8 g, Sugars: 0.3 g, Protein: 2.1 g

Apple Pie Crackers

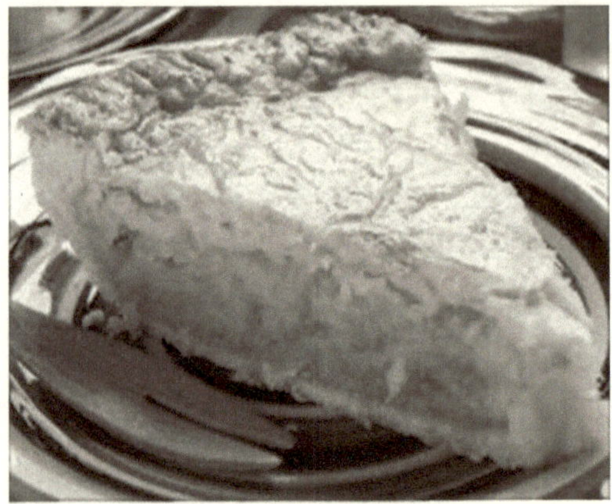

Serves: 100 crackers

Ingredients:

- 2 Tbsp + 2 tsp Avocado Oil

- 1 medium Granny Smith Apple, roughly chopped

- ¼ cup Erythritol

- ¼ cup Sunflower Seeds, finely ground

- 1¾ cup Roughly Ground Flax Seed

- 1/8 tsp Ground Cloves

- 1/8 tsp Ground Cardamom

- 3 Tbsp Ground Cinnamon

- ¼ tsp Ground Nutmeg

- ¼ tsp Ground Ginger

Directions:

- Preheat your oven to 225F / 110C. Line two baking sheets with parchment paper and set them aside.

- Combine the oil, apple, and erythritol in your food processor, add the remaining ingredients and blend until well combined.

- Transfer the batter to your prepared baking sheets, spread evenly and cut into crackers.

- Bake in the preheated oven for an hour. Flip the crackers, remove the parchment paper and continue baking for one more hour. If the crackers are thick, they will need more time to bake.

- When done, leave to cool and serve.

Nutrients per one serving:

Calories: 11.5, Total Fat: 2.1 g, Saturated Fat: 0.2 g, Carbs: 0.9 g, Sugars: 0 g, Protein: 0.4 g

Crispy Almond Crackers

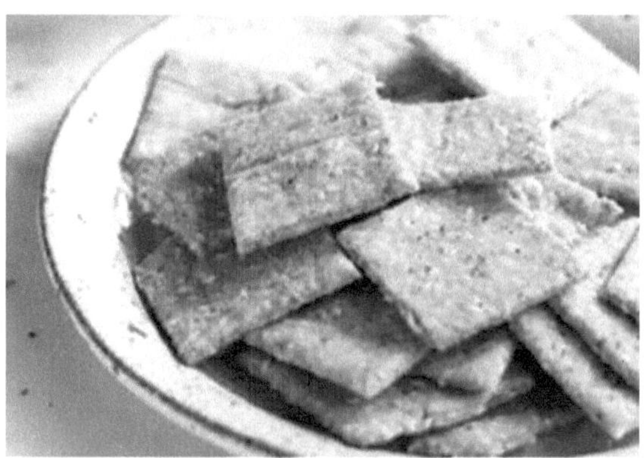

Serves: 40 crackers

Ingredients:

- 1 cup Almond Flour

- 1/4 tsp Baking Soda

- 1/4 tsp Salt

- 1/8 tsp Black Pepper

- 3 Tbsp Sesame Seeds

- 1 Egg, beaten

- Salt and Black Pepper, to top the crackers

Directions:

- Preheat your oven to 350F / 175C. Line two baking sheets with parchment paper and set aside.

- Mix all the dry ingredients to a large bowl. Add the egg and mix well to incorporate and form a dough. Divide the dough into two balls.

- Roll out the dough between two pieces of parchment paper. Cut into crackers and transfer them to the prepared baking sheet.

- Bake for about 15-20 minutes. In the meantime, repeat the same procedure with the remaining dough.

- Once done, leave the crackers to cool and serve.

Nutrients per one serving:

Calories: 21.7, Total Fat: 2.9 g, Saturated Fat: 0.2 g, Carbs: 0.8 g, Sugars: 0.1 g, Protein: 0.9 g

Easy Sesame Breadsticks

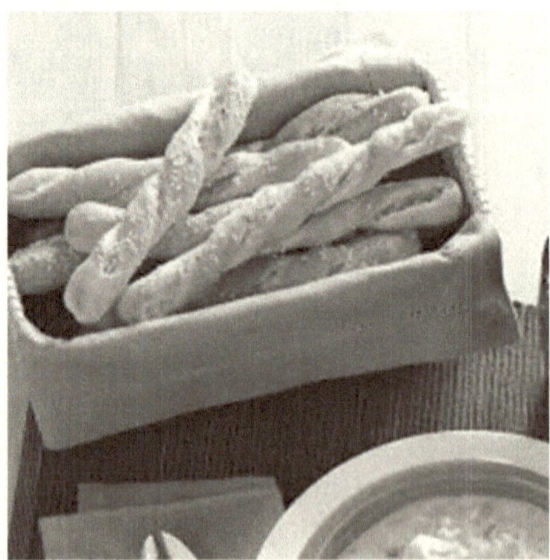

Serves: 5 breadsticks

Ingredients:

- 1 Egg White

- 2 Tbsp Almond Flour

- 1 tsp Himalayan Pink Salt

- 1 Tbsp Extra Virgin Olive Oil

- ½ tsp Sesame Seeds

Directions:

- Preheat your oven to 320F / 160C. Line a baking sheet with parchment paper and set aside.

- Whisk the egg white and add the flour as well as half each the salt and olive oil.

- Knead until you get a smooth dough, divide into 5 pieces and roll into breadsticks.

- Place on the prepared sheet, brush with the remaining olive oil and sprinkle with the sesame seeds and the remaining salt.

- Bake for about 20 minutes. Allow cooling slightly before serving.

Nutrients per one serving:

Calories: 53.6, Total Fat: 5 g, Saturated Fat: 0.6 g, Carbs: 1.1 g, Sugars: 0.2 g, Protein: 1.6 g

Salty Rosemary Crackers

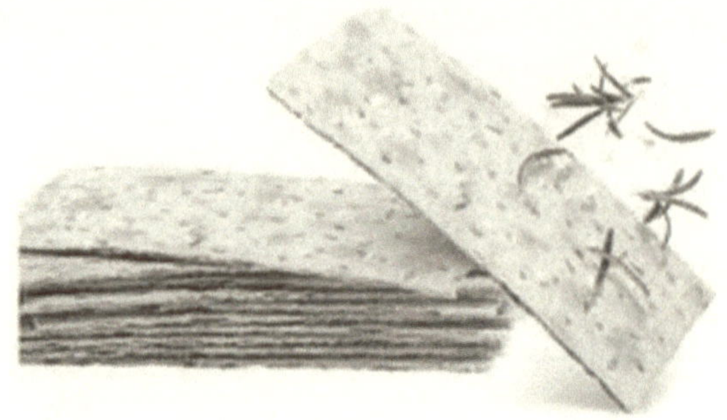

Serves: 36 crackers

Ingredients:

*   1 1/2 cup Almond Flour

*   1/2 tsp Celtic Sea Salt

*   1 Egg, room temperature

*   2 Tbsp Coconut Oil

*   1/4 tsp Black Pepper

*   1 Tbsp Finely Chopped Rosemary

Directions:

*   Preheat your oven to 350F / 175C. Line a baking tray with parchment paper and set aside.

*   Mix together the almond flour and salt and set aside.

*   In another bowl, whisk together the egg, coconut oil, black pepper, and rosemary. Add the mixture to the almond flour mixture and mix well until dough forms.

*   Transfer the dough to a piece of parchment paper, cover with another piece and roll it out into a thin layer. Cut into crackers, arrange them on the

prepared sheet and bake for about 10-15 minutes.

- Allow cooling when done and to serve.

Nutrients per one serving:

Calories: 35.2, Total Fat: 5.2 g, Saturated Fat: 1.9 g, Carbs: 1 g, Sugars: 0.2 g, Protein: 1.2 g

Onion & Thyme Cracker

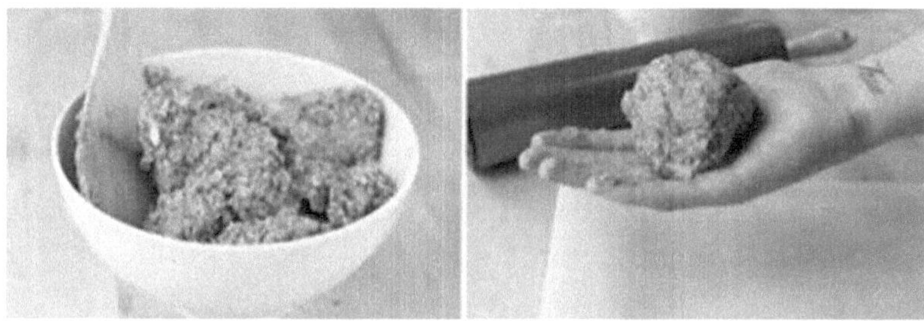

Serves: 75 crackers

Ingredients:

- 1 Garlic Clove, minced

- 1 cup Coarsely Chopped Sweet Onion

- 2 tsp Fresh Thyme Leaves

- ¼ cup Avocado Oil

- ¼ tsp Himalayan Salt

- Freshly Ground Pepper, to taste

- ¼ cup Sunflower Seeds

- 1½ cups Roughly Ground Flax Seeds

Directions:

- Preheat your oven to 225F / 110C. Line two baking sheets with parchment paper and set aside.

- Combine the garlic, onion, thyme, oil, salt, and pepper in your food processor. Add the sunflower and flax seeds and pulse until completely pureed.

- Transfer the batter to your prepared baking sheets and spread it evenly and cut into crackers.

- Bake for an hour, remove the parchment paper, flip the crackers and continue baking for another hour. If the crackers are thick, it will take them more time to bake.

- Once done, remove from the oven, allow to cool and serve.

Nutrients per one serving:

Calories: 18, Total Fat: 2.7 g, Saturated Fat: 0.2 g, Carbs: 0.8 g, Sugars: 0.3 g, Protein: 0.4 g

Pretzel-like Crackers

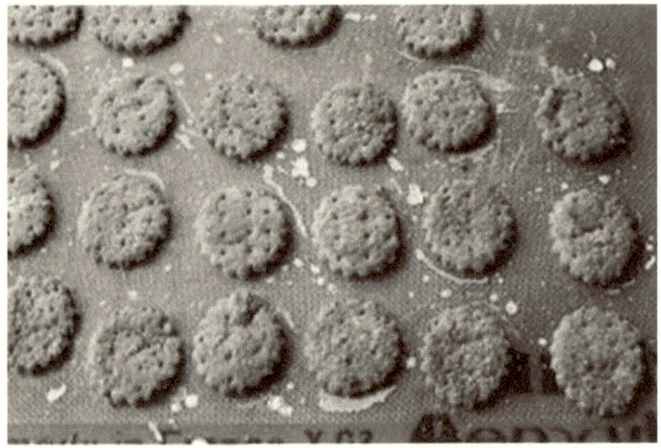

Serves: 15 crackers

Ingredients:

1/2 cup Ghee

1/2 cup Water

- 2 Tbsp Apple Cider Vinegar

- 1/2 tsp Sea Salt

- 1/2 cup Tapioca Flour

- 1/2 tsp Baking Powder

- 1/2 tsp Baking Soda

- 1 Egg

- 1 cup Coconut Flour

Directions:

- Preheat your oven to 350F / 175C. Line a baking sheet with parchment paper and set aside.

- Add the ghee, water, vinegar, and salt to a saucepan and bring to the boil over medium heat.

- Once it starts boiling, remove from the heat and stir in the tapioca flour. Add the baking powder and soda and mix for about 3-5 seconds as the mixture foams.

- Add the egg and coconut flour and mix until dough forms.

- Knead the dough for a minute or two and then divide into small balls. Roll each ball into a log and twist it into a pretzel shape.

- Arrange on the prepared baking sheet and bake for about half an hour.

- Allow cooling slightly before serving.

Nutrients per one serving:

Calories: 92.2, Total Fat: 10.2 g, Saturated Fat: 2.1 g, Carbs: 4.5 g, Sugars: 0 g, Protein: 1.4 g

Basil & Oregano Breadsticks

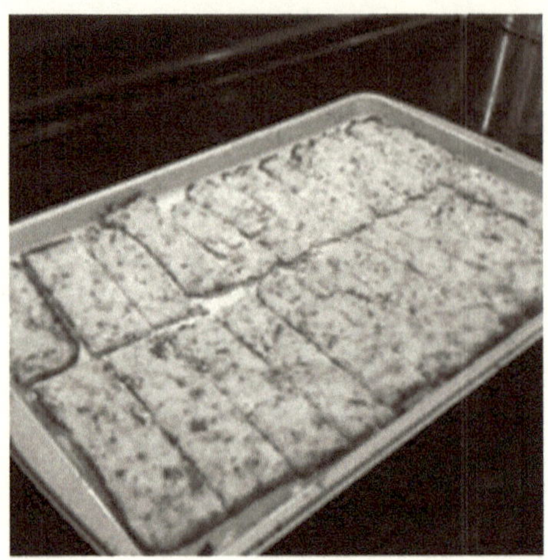

Serves: 4-8 breadsticks

Ingredients:

- 3 Eggs, divided

- 1 1/3 cup Almond Flour

- 2 Tbsp Coconut Oil, melted

- 1/2 tsp Baking Powder

- 1/2 tsp Salt

- 3 Tbsp Coconut Flour

- 1/2 tsp Oregano

- 1 tsp Dried Basil

- 1 Garlic Clove, minced

- 1/2 tsp Onion Powder

- Ghee, for brushing

Directions:

• Preheat your oven to 350F / 175C. Line a baking sheet with parchment paper and set aside.

• Whisk two eggs and set aside.

• In another bowl, combine the almond flour, coconut oil, baking powder, and salt. Add the beaten eggs and mix well to combine.

• Add 1 tbsp coconut flour and give the dough a minute to absorb it. Repeat with the remaining flour and knead the mixture into smooth dough.

• Roll out the dough onto a piece of parchment paper and form breadsticks. Place on the preheated sheet and bake for about 10 minutes.

• Whisk the remaining egg and use it to brush the breadsticks. Sprinkle them with the oregano, basil, minced garlic, and onion powder and return to the oven to bake for 5 more minutes.

• Once baked, brush with some melted ghee, serve warm or allow to cool.

Nutrients per one serving:

Calories: 322, Total Fat: 28.4 g, Saturated Fat: 7.4 g, Carbs: 12 g, Sugars: 1.5 g, Protein: 9.8 g

Simple Keto Breadsticks

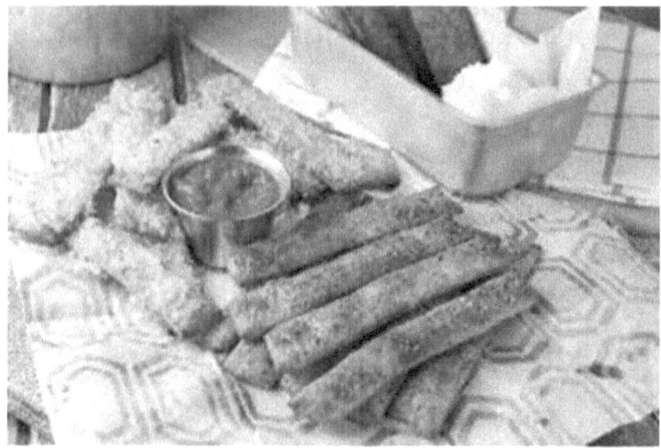

Serves: 8

Ingredients:

- 1/3 cup Coconut Flour

- 1/3 cup Arrowroot Flour

- 1/2 tsp Baking Soda

- 1 1/2 tsp Lemon Juice

- 1 tsp Dried Rosemary

- 3 Tbsp Water

- 1 Egg

- 4 Tbsp Extra Virgin Olive Oil, divided use - 3 Tbsp for breadsticks, 1 Tbsp for topping

- 1/8 tsp Garlic Powder, for topping

- 1/8 tsp Sea Salt, for topping

Directions:

- Preheat your oven to 350F / 175C. Line a baking sheet with parchment paper and set aside.

- Add all the ingredients to your food processor and pulse until well combined and the dough is formed.

- Divide the dough into 8 equal balls and roll them into breadsticks. Arrange on the prepared sheet, brush with olive oil and sprinkle with the garlic powered and salt.

- Bake for about 10 minutes and serve warm or allow to cool.

Nutrients per one serving:

Calories: 216, Total Fat: 15.8 g, Saturated Fat: 2.2 g, Carbs: 8.1 g, Sugars: 0.1 g, Protein: 3.1 g

Ultimate Keto Breadsticks

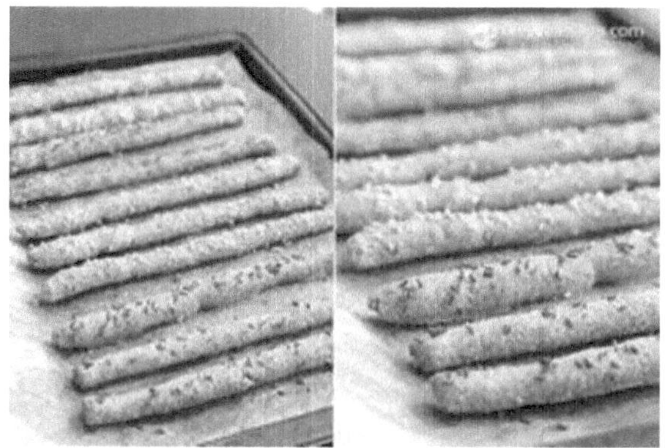

Serves: 20 breadsticks

Ingredients:

- ¼ cup Coconut Flour

- ¾ cup Ground Flax Seeds

- 1 Tbsp Psyllium Husk Powder

- 1 cup Almond Flour

- 2 Tbsp Ground Chia Seeds

- 1 tsp Salt

- 1 cup Lukewarm Water, plus more if the dough is too dry

Ingredients for the topping:

- 2 Egg Yolks, for brushing

- 4 Tbsp Mixed Seeds

- 1 tsp Coarse Sea Salt

Directions:

- Combine the coconut flour, flax seeds, psyllium husks, and almond flour. Add the chia seeds, salt, and the water. Mix until dough is formed.

Refrigerate for about 20 minutes.

•	In the meantime, preheat your oven to 350F / 175C. Line a baking sheet with parchment paper and set aside.

•	Divide the dough into 20 equal pieces and roll them with your hands forming breadsticks.

•	Arrange the breadsticks on the baking sheet and brush them with the egg yolks.

•	Sprinkle with seeds and salt and bake for about 20 minutes.

•	Serve warm or allow to cool.

Nutrients per one serving:

Calories: 75.2, Total Fat: 9.6 g, Saturated Fat: 1.5 g, Carbs: 4.1 g, Sugars: 0.2 g, Protein: 3.5 g.

Conclusion

Many simple sweet and savory fat bombs from the available products will make your food system more effective. If you decide to receive amazing results of weight loss on a ketogenic diet, so fat bombs will help you to master it more easily.

Since fat bombs are an important part of our daily and special cuisines, nobody wants to miss out their mouth-pleasing flavors just because they are on a ketogenic diet plan. This cookbook brings comfort and ease to such minds and discusses the basic of ketogenic diet combined with the idea of fat bombs and then unveils few of the delicious recipes that every keto dieter can try at home without worries. So, every time you make your mind to try a quick snack or make an energy boosting breakfast or to experiment with a dessert, this cookbook is here to help you through the process.

-SANDRA M.-

CHECK OUT OTHER BOOKS

Go here to check out other related books that might interest you:

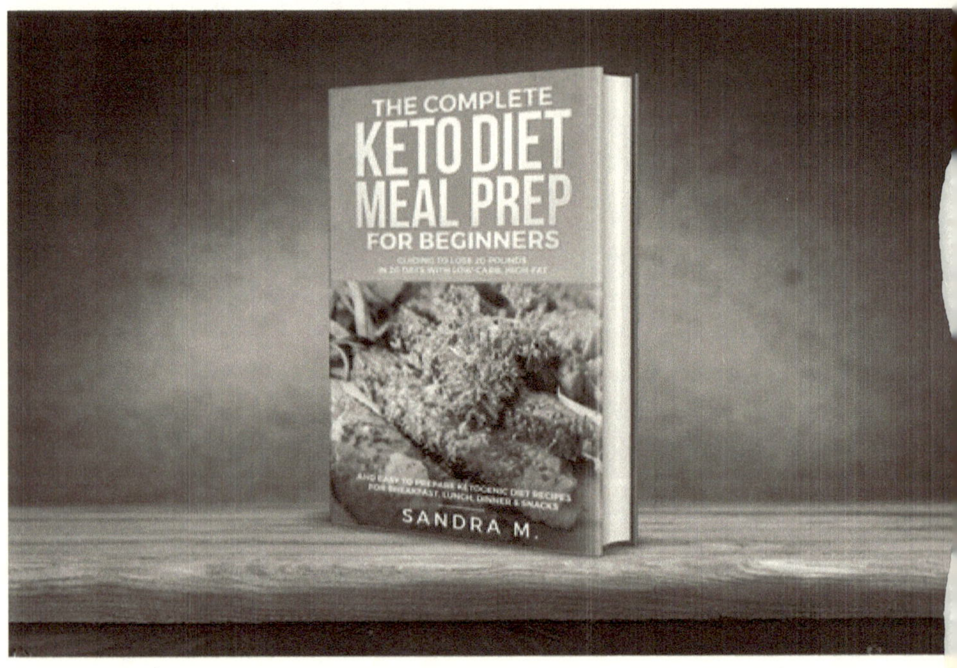

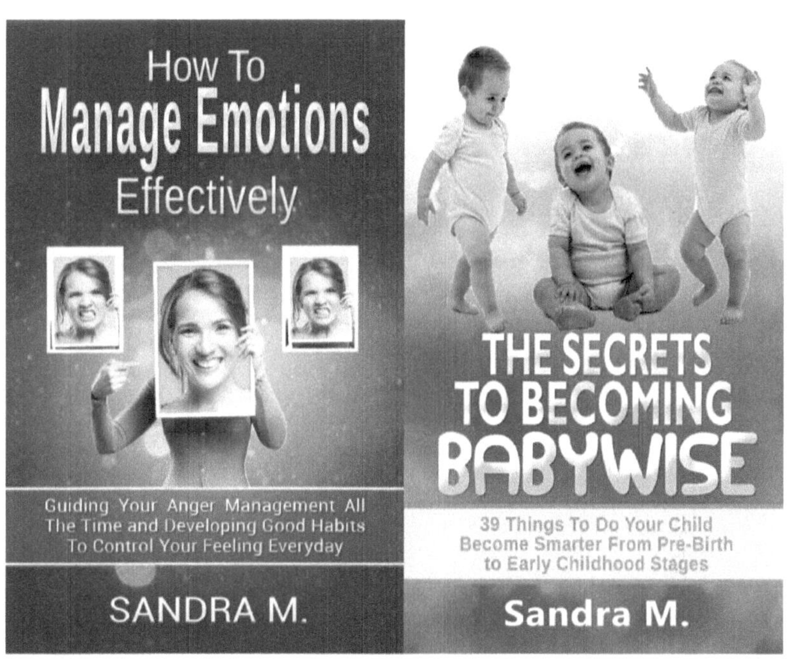
How To
Manage Emotions
Effectively

Guiding Your Anger Management All
The Time and Developing Good Habits
To Control Your Feeling Everyday

SANDRA M.

THE SECRETS
TO BECOMING
BABYWISE

39 Things To Do Your Child
Become Smarter From Pre-Birth
to Early Childhood Stages

Sandra M.

9 781792 828225